After BSE – A future for the European livestock sector

The EAAP series is published under the direction of Dr. P. Rafai

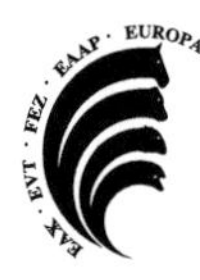

EAAP – European Association for Animal Production

The European Association for Animal Production wishes to express its appreciation to the *Ministero per le Politiche Agricole e Forestali* and the *Associazione Italiana Allevatori* for their valuable support of its activities

After BSE – A future for the European livestock sector

EAAP publication No. 108

Editor

E.P. Cunningham

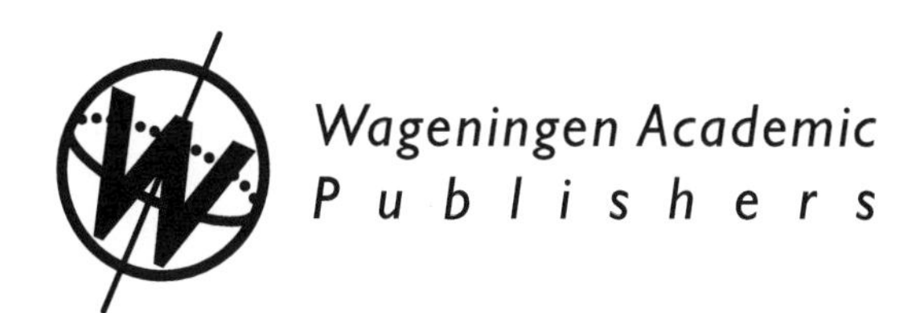

CIP-data Koninklijke Bibliotheek, Den Haag

ISBN 907699823X paperback
ISSN 0071-2477
NUGI 835

Subject headings:
BSE epidemic
Food chain
Future options

First published, 2003

Wageningen Academic Publishers
The Netherlands, 2003

Table of contents

Page

Preface

Europe faced a major crisis over the BSE phenomenon. In addition to affecting cattle breeders and beef producers the BSE crisis involved many other sectors of society. These include the associated activities of animal health, meat processing, leather industry, wholesale and retail sale of beef, national and international trade, movement control of farm animals and, last but not least, the perceived new threat to human health by CJD with all its complex interactions between science, medicine, politics and legislation. This crisis had also other effects such as declining public confidence in science, a lack of trust in official and other official supervision of issues affecting human health, broken farm businesses, a growing cost to governments and to the EU; necessary actions to limit the spread of BSE into further countries and territories.

The long term effect and the ultimate impact of BSE on human society is still not fully clear and future livestock production and animal health practices are still being debated. The way forward needs to be further clarified.

EAAP proposed therefore to prepare a comprehensive Report on BSE which draws upon the deep strengths of the Association in the livestock sector in all its components. The aim of the Report is not to defend the sectional interests of animal production. Rather it seeks to provide light for those in all sectors of society who have to make decisions on this difficult topic and in the future beware of other eventual emergencies. Therefore the composition of the Group established by EAAP to produce the Report includes, along with livestock scientists, distinguished experts from other sectors such as consumer concerns, trade, economics and health.

The outcome is a balanced, objective and forward-looking report which seeks to provide new perspectives and some options for the future, based upon a full understanding of the past. The Report had not the purpose of documenting again the causes of BSE nor to gainsay the scientific information already published by recognized and authoritative bodies dealing with the animal health issues.

It was appropriate that the EAAP, with its clear mandate for Animal Science and Production in Europe and the Mediterranean basin, should offer a comprehensive view on the difficult issues that our society faced at large and should seek to identify realistic and creative ways to overcome the existing problems with some indication of how to prevent a recurrence of similar situations in the future.

We want to thank Patrick Cunningham and his team for taking on this difficult assignment and successfully proposing a view of the needs of the livestock sector of tomorrow: animal health monitoring, animal products risk assessment and better animal agriculture management but also and above all food security, the consumers' awareness of food quality, professional ethics in the livestock sector and the animals' welfare.

Aimé Aumaitre
(President EAAP) and

Jean Boyazoglu
(Executive Vice-President EAAP)

Paris, June 2003

After BSE - A future for the European Livestock Sector

Introduction

When, on March 20th, 1996, the UK government announced its belief in a probable link between the brain disease BSE in cattle and the similar disease vCJD in humans, an unprecedented crisis struck the beef production sector in Europe.

The crisis was first, and most dramatically, a crisis of confidence. Consumers reacted instantly by taking their business elsewhere. As the continuing publicity has highlighted various related and unrelated deficiencies in the production chain, there has been permanent damage to the relationship between consumers and producers. Secondly, there was an economic crisis, mainly borne by producers. The scale of the economic loss has been much greater than is generally appreciated. Like the impact on consumer confidence, these economic effects will continue into the future. Thirdly, there was a crisis for the public authorities. Large and unbudgeted costs were incurred. Regulatory structures were shown to be inadequate. The result has been a rapid restructuring of public services in areas of agriculture, food and public health in all European counties, and at EU level.

This multiple crisis occurred in an industry already struggling to adapt to the demands of changing consumer requirements, increasing competition, declining profitability, and advancing technology. In the years to come, these parallel challenges are likely to be intensified.

At an early stage in the BSE crisis EAAP has already issued a special publication on the disease and its implications (EAAP, 1994). It also commissioned a major study on the future evolution of the livestock sector (Politiek and Bakker, 1982). The purpose of the present report is to carry forward that work: to document the lessons learnt from the rolling BSE crisis, and to consider the future evolution of the livestock sector in Europe.

The Working Group

Juan José Badiola (Spain)
Gottfried Brem (Germany)
Fernando Crespo (OIE)
Patrick Cunningham (Ireland, Chairman)
Jean-Claude Flamant (France)
Janet Graham (UK)
John Hodges (Austria)
Karsten Klint Jensen (Denmark)
Samuel Jutzi (FAO)
François Madec (France, Secretary)
Ben Mepham (UK)
Attila Nagy (Hungary)
Alessandro Nardone (Italy)
Peter Sandoe (Denmark)

Acknowledgements

The European Association for Animal Production (EAAP) wants to acknowledge the meaningful technical inputs and support received from the FAO (AGA) and OIE during various stages of this project's development. EAAP wants also to express its great appreciation to the Italian Ministry of Agricultural and Forestry Policies (MiPAF) and the FAO for their important financial participation.

Executive Summary

- The BSE epidemic, which began in 1986, is now gradually coming to an end. Though knowledge is incomplete, enough is known about the disease to be reasonably confident that such an epidemic will not recur.

- Three principal questions remain unresolved: the origin of the BSE epidemic; the future of vCJD; and what to do with the 16 million tonnes of animal byproducts produced annually by the slaughter industry.

- Loss of value and cost of disposal of MBM exceed 1.5 billion Euro per year. Though new EU legislation could permit over 80% of this material to be used again in livestock feeds, the best option is to continue the ban on its use.

- The cost of the epidemic has been enormous, and is estimated here at about 10% of the annual output value of the European beef sector. The discounted present value of these costs is estimated at €92 billion.

- The progress of the epidemic was marked by many deficiencies and failures, of which two are particularly noted.
  - The inadequacies of public information, particularly in the UK
  - Failure to prevent international spread through contaminated meat and bone meal.

- Ongoing changes in the industry are documented: changing consumer requirements; concentration of processing and retailing power; declining producer prices, and reduction in numbers of full time producers. These changes represent both the causes and effects of a continuing shift in the terms of trade to the disadvantage of producers. To ensure fair trading, increased controls to prevent abuse of economic power may be necessary.

- The ten countries which are destined to join the EU have 40% more farmers than in the EU 15. The challenge of accommodating them in a common EU policy, market and budget has major implications for the existing EU livestock sector.

- European production costs for milk, red meats and cereals (the raw material for white meat production) are higher than in the traditional exporting countries for these commodities. This is partly due to relative scales of production units. With progressive trade liberalisation, continued pressure on producer prices is inevitable.

- Steady increases in unit scale and intensification, particularly in pig, poultry and dairy enterprises, have generated problems of nutrient overload in some regions. The industry will need to acknowledge and address these problems.

- In the present context it is ironic to note that the situation on animal disease in Europe has never been better. All major diseases are eradicated or under control. For the future the emphasis will be on the control of enzootic diseases, largely through husbandry practices; reduction, and eventual elimination of routine use of antibiotics in feeds; and intensive research to cope with emerging diseases.

- Scientists have lost credibility as a result of the BSE crisis. While it is more critical than ever that public policy be informed by the best scientific advice, those involved in providing such advice must more carefully identify and distinguish the factual basis from the value judgements involved.

- Scientific innovation has also lost favour with the public, particularly where it affects food and health. The livestock sector will need to weigh carefully the technical benefits against the risks and public acceptability of technologies such as GMOs, BST in milk production, growth promoters in meat production.

- Given that over 95% of European livestock production is destined for European consumers, the production industry must concentrate on securing their loyalty by fulfilling their expectations on
  - food safety;
  - transparency and accountability;
  - quality and variety, including response to the demand for regional and organic products.

- New ways need to be found to build the community of interest of producers, processors, and retailers in meeting these goals.

Chapter 1. BSE: the Facts, the Impact, the Lessons

1.1 The Epidemic in the UK

The cattle disease now known as Bovine Spongiform Encephalopathy (BSE) was first confirmed in a cow on a dairy farm in the south of England in 1985. It is believed that unrecorded cases had occurred earlier than this. The disease, occurring in both sexes in adult animals, is a neurological condition involving pronounced changes in mental state, abnormalities of posture, movement and sensation. Symptoms characteristically last for several weeks and are progressive and fatal. Post-mortem examination of bovine brain demonstrated similar pathology to the family of Transmissible Spongiform Encephalopathies (TSEs), a group of diseases occurring in several mammalian species and in humans. The new disease became known as Bovine Spongiform Encephalopathy (BSE), a form of TSE thought at the time to be specific to cattle.

In the years following 1986, the number of cases in the UK increased dramatically, peaking at 37,289 cases in 1992. Since then, the epidemic has declined steadily, and the number of cases reported in the UK in 2002 was 1144. While the disease has spread to other countries, over 95% of all recorded cases to date have occurred in the UK. The course of the epidemic in that country and the parallel actions taken are shown in **Figure 1.1**.

In 1988 the disease was declared a zoonosis, an infectious disease transmissible under natural conditions from vertebrate animals to man. This was noteworthy as conventional wisdom until then held that the disease was species-specific and posed no danger to human health. The confirmation, in 1997, that BSE was no longer confined solely to cattle, but was the probable cause of new variant Creutzfeldt-Jakob Disease (vCJD) in humans was a most significant event (Bruce *et al.* 1997, Hill *et al.* 1997). The first case of human vCJD was detected in the UK in 1994, and by 2002 over 100 cases had been recorded. This threat to human health has led to the implementation of a number of critical response measures.

The origins, progress and eventual control of BSE in the UK are marked by a number of crucial advances in knowledge and consequential responses. Initial epidemiological analysis showed the pattern of BSE cases to be typical of an epidemic involving many individual, independent disease outbreaks, each of which could be traced to a common source. The only common feature of all investigated cases was the use of commercially produced compound feed containing meat and bone meal (MBM) (Wilesmith *et al.* 1988). Following the understanding that MBM was the probable medium for spread of the disease (Southwood, 1989) progressive measures were established to eliminate infectious material from MBM and to remove MBM from animal feed. In July 1988 ruminant MBM was banned specifically from ruminant feed and later (1996) from all animal rations. Meanwhile specified risk material (SRM), including ruminant offal and brain, was excluded from human consumption and animal feed and was banned from export from the UK. By 1995 regulations on mechanically recovered meat (MRM) were also introduced.

These measures, increasingly effective in the UK, resulted in the displacement of MBM from the UK market. This led to an increase in export of MBM, initially to EU countries,

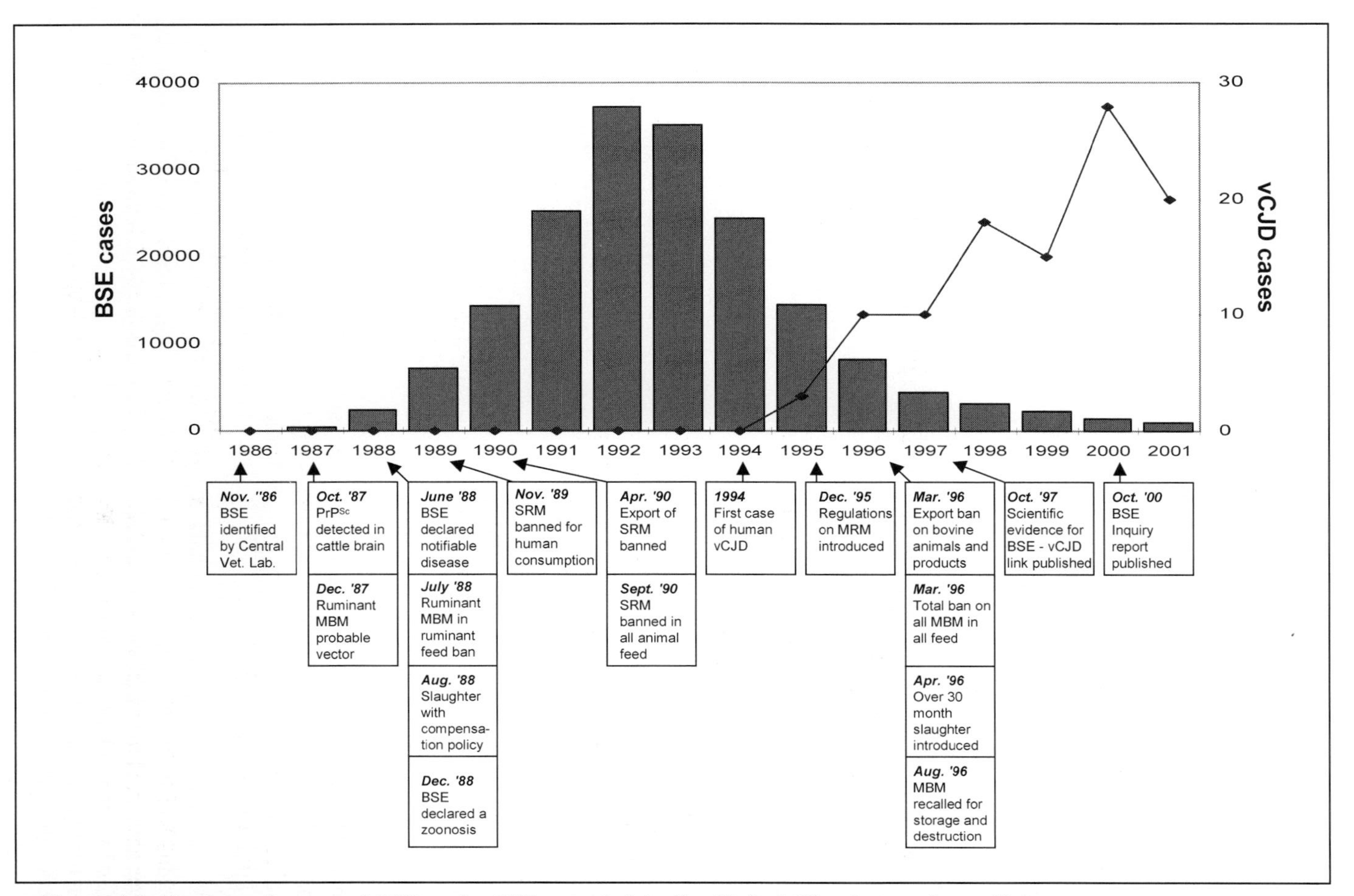

Figure 1.1 Number of cases of BSE and vCJD reported in the United Kingdom and parallel response measures (Sources: OIE, DEFRA).

and as its use was banned there, to more distant markets. In August 1996 all MBM in the UK was recalled for storage and destruction.

As research and field experience produced new information on the nature of the disease, containment and eradication measures were steadily increased. These have been largely successful in preventing new infections in the cattle population. This is confirmed by the fact that, almost without exception, all newly recorded cases are in animals born before 1996.

The success of the measures taken to prevent infected animals entering the human food chain is not yet clear. Numbers of vCJD cases have shown a rising trend since 1994. A number of uncertainties (exposure/dose, susceptibility, incubation period) mean that accurate prediction of future numbers is difficult. Most estimates put the total number of expected cases between a few hundred and several thousand, though under some sets of assumptions, total expected cases could exceed 100 000 (POST 2002, Valleron *et al.* 2001, d'Aigneaux *et al.* 2001, Ghani *et al.* 2000, Ferguson *et al.* 2002).

The epidemic has had catastrophic economic consequences for UK farms, and for the economy. Real producer prices for beef fell dramatically in 1989 and in 1996 in response to waves of concern for the safety of the product (**Figure 1.2**). Economic loss to the UK in the year following the 1996 crisis was estimated at €1.2 - 1.6 billion, or between 62% and 82% of the total farm gate value of beef output. The cumulative budgetary cost of BSE since 1996 was estimated to reach €5.6 billion by the end of 2001 (Atkinson 2001).

About one half to two thirds of the national loss was accounted for by the fall in the value added of meat production. The remainder resulted from the cost of operating the various public schemes, compliance costs associated with new legislative requirements and costs associated with the adjustments of production to service new markets. The impact on specific sectors varied. For example, in the first year the beef producers were largely protected from the crisis by various compensation payments. Slaughterers and renderers also benefited from the various schemes introduced during the crisis. On the other hand, meat manufacturers and retailers received no compensation, but the larger businesses were able to adjust their product mix.

1.2 International Spread

Some years after the BSE epidemic was established in the UK, cases began to occur in other countries. Beginning with Ireland (1989) the disease has now been reported in some 19 additional countries, most of them in Europe (**Table 1.1**). In most countries the numbers of cases are very small, and were it not for the increased vigilance would possibly have gone unnoticed. In all cases, containment measures are in place such that any threat to animal or human health is controlled.

In each country where BSE has occurred, there have been two critical points. The first is the recognition that BSE exists in the national cattle herd. The second is the confirmation of vCJD in the human population. These events have occurred at different times in different countries (Table 1.1). Each event has provoked a crisis of public confidence in food safety and in the national regulatory agencies, with severe effects on economic life.

Each country has developed a set of responses to these crises. In addition, the EU has taken actions applicable across countries. These responses have evolved progressively as knowledge of the two diseases has increased.

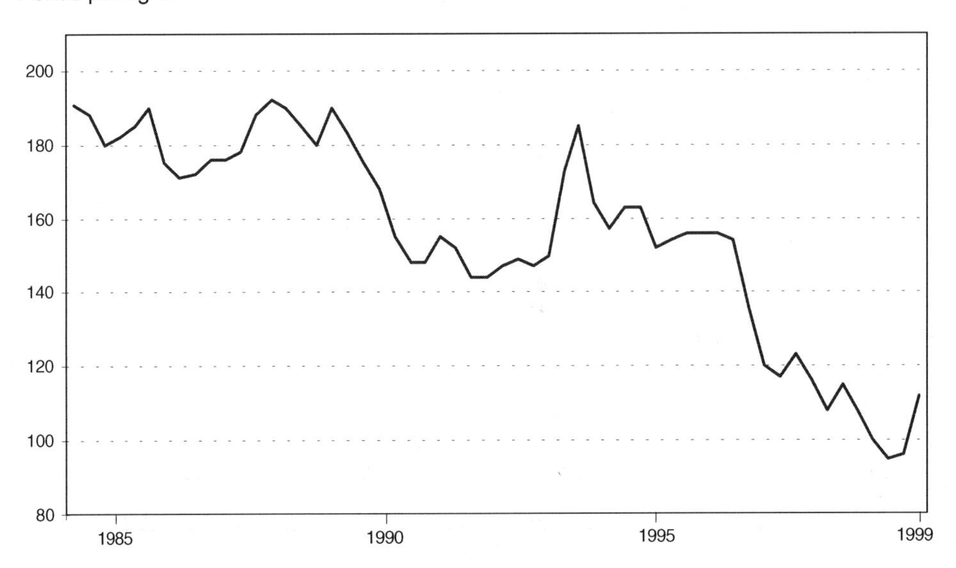

Figure 1.2. UK real beef producer prices (January 1987 money). (Source: Atkinson, 2001).

Table 1.1 BSE, vCJD incidence and total cattle population in selected countries. Figures are to January 2002. (Sources: DEFRA, OIE & FAO).

	Total BSE cases	Date of first incidence	Total vCJD cases	Total cattle population (heads)
United Kingdom	181 375	1986	106	10 598 000
Ireland	833	1989	1	6 459 300
Portugal	628	1990		1 250 000
Switzerland	403	1990		1 610 800
France	499	1991	4	20 500 000
Denmark	8	1992		1 850 000
Germany	152	1992		14 480 000
Italy	54	1994	1	7 211 000
Belgium	68	1997		3 040 000
Luxembourg	1	1997		205 000
Liechtenstein	2	1998		6 000
The Netherlands	28	1997		4 050 000
Spain	88	2000		6 163 900
Austria	1	2001		2 155 447
Czech Rep.	2	2001		1 582 027
Finland	1	2001		1 085 000
Greece	1	2001		585 000
Japan	3	2001		4 530 000
Slovakia	5	2001		646 100
Slovenia	1	2001		493 670

1.3 Cost of the Epidemic

For most animal disease outbreaks (for example FMD - see **Box 4**), the costs of containment, eradication and economic adjustment are temporary. After the outbreak has been brought under control, the industry returns to normal. BSE has been different. New and permanent changes have been introduced which impose substantial additional costs for the indefinite future.

The cost of the BSE epidemic has varied from country to country with the incidence of cases and with the different policies applied. The UK had by far the largest number of cases, but adopted a policy of slaughtering only affected animals, on the grounds that lateral transmission was not believed to occur. Other countries, with fewer cases, slaughtered the whole herd where an affected animal was found. This was regarded as a reasonable precautionary measure given a degree of uncertainty about the nature of transmission, and to secure public confidence in the containment measures.

However, the largest cost is not involved in control measures, but in the permanent loss in value of each beef animal produced due to the exclusion from the food chain of certain carcass components. In addition, new costs per animal are incurred for the safe disposal of waste material, for animal testing, and for extra procedures and precautions in the slaughtering industry. A set of estimates of these losses and costs is given in **Box 1**.

What is the total cost of the BSE epidemic in the EU? From the figures in Box 1, it is clear that a figure varying around €100 per animal is involved. Over half of this is the loss in carcass value, and the remainder consists of Meat and Bone Meal (MBM) disposal, depopulation of affected herds, and BSE testing costs. The average value of all bovines slaughtered in the EU is close to €1000. Thus, about 10% of the value of each beef animal produced has been lost.

Irrespective of the future course of the epidemic, most of this loss in value per animal will continue. Some MBM use might be resumed, and BSE testing costs might be reduced. However, the changes in meat industry practices will be permanent. Furthermore, the calculations given here take no account of the costs associated with vCJD in humans, nor of the impact of BSE on beef prices at retail level. The figure of 10% of the value of beef output is therefore a reasonable starting point from which to estimate the economic impact in the EU.

In 2000, beef accounted for 10.2% of the total value of agricultural output in the EU, or €27.5 bn. The annual loss as a result of BSE can therefore be estimated approximately as 10% of this, or €2.75 bn. Discounting all future losses this gives a Net Present Value (NPV) of approximately A/r, where A is the annual loss and r is the discount rate. With an annual loss of A = €2.75 bn and a discount rate of r = 0.03, this gives a NPV of €92 bn.

This is an enormous sum, approximately equal to the whole annual budget of the EU. Higher discount rates or a shorter time horizon would produce lower estimates. However, no reasonable recalculation is likely to reduce this estimate by 50%. Even if, as is expected, the BSE epidemic in Europe is coming to an end, its economic shock effect on the livestock sector has been immense.

1.4 The Learning Curve

The BSE epidemic is perhaps unique in the 20th century in the degree of ignorance of its causes and nature at the time of the outbreak. While a number of TSEs (the most relevant and notable being scrapie in sheep) were

Box 1. BSE Impact on Animal Value

Before BSE became part of the cattle industry, every element of an animal presented for slaughter had value. The bulk of the carcass went into the human food chain. Meat waste and trim went to the pet food market. Fat trim was rendered for a variety of food and industrial end uses. Bone was processed into meat and bone meal for the livestock feed industry.
Post BSE, the destiny and value of many of these components has changed. In many cases components which could previously have been sold must now be disposed of. Instead of contributing to value, they have therefore contributed additional cost.
It is difficult to quantify this change in the values and costs at an industry level. No comprehensive figures are collected. In addition, there are considerable differences between countries in the average slaughter weight of animals, and in the traditional use patterns of the components of the slaughter animal. It is, however, possible to illustrate the change in values and costs in particular cases, and these can give a general sense of the more widespread pattern of change. Table 1 shows the values and costs in 1995 and in 2002 at one substantial beef slaughter plant.

Table 1 Component costs and values of beef animal pre and post BSE.

	Value euro / head		
	Pre BSE	Post BSE	Difference
Edible offals	10.09	2.72	7.37
Inedible offals	4.45	-2.74	7.19
Fat	11.13	1.02	10.11
Bone	3.39	-2.36	5.75
SRM	0.00	-12.11	12.11
MRM	6.00	0.00	6.00
Increased labour: cost per head			1.92
Reduced processing rate: cost per head			4.70
Total revenue loss per head			55.15

The amount of useable fat has gone down greatly, with a loss in value of €10.11 per head. Bone, pre BSE, included nearly all the material which is now classified as specified risk (SRM). Today, the SRM is separately treated. The amount of SRM per head has increased steadily as the definition has been broadened to include additional materials, and now accounts for some 40 - 50 kgs, depending on the weight of the animal. On average, in this plant, it has a disposal cost of €12.11 per head. Edible offals have been reduced in value by €7.37 per head and inedible offals by €7.17. Finally, mechanically recovered meat (MRM), which formerly had a value of €6.00 per head, now has zero value. The total revenue loss per head from the change in value of these components amounts to €48.53 per animal.
With the increased segregation of materials necessary in a meat plant to cope with BSE precautions, substantial changes in work practices have been necessary. In this plant an additional five workstations were required. In addition, the rate of throughput on the slaughter line is reduced, thereby increasing operating costs. These additional costs amount to €6.62 per head, bringing the total reduction in revenue per head to €55.15.
These estimates should be regarded as establishing the minimum impact of BSE on the value at slaughter of a beef animal. To implement the new regulations additional capital expenditure has been incurred throughout the beef industry. In addition, the rendering, storage and destruction of meat and bone meal has been subsidised to the extent of €670 per tonne, or €21.45 per animal. Futher control measures require a BSE test for animals over 30 months to enter the market. Otherwise they are purchased for destruction. Herds with affected animals are depopulated with compensation. Averaged over all cattle slaughtered, these additional costs come to €27.68 per head. The total estimated cost per head therefore amounts to €104.28, or about 10 % of the value of the animal.

known, their causative agent was a mystery. The pattern of transmission was also mysterious, and no effective treatment was known.

The key scientific advance was the discovery in 1986 that the infective agent of BSE was an aberrant form of a normal class of protein called prions (Prusiner 1986, 1987). Furthermore, it was found that the aberrant form could induce structural changes in normal prions, converting them to the pathological form. The presence of these pathological prions in brain tissue gives rise to irreversible changes leading to the symptoms of the disease.

Further research showed that the disease could be established in several species (mice, calves, sheep, goats, mink) by injection or ingestion of the aberrant prion. Since the occurrence of the first recorded case of vCJD in 1994, cumulative scientific evidence points to ingestion of aberrant prions, probably of bovine origin, as the likely cause (Bruce *et al.* 1997).

Research has also shown that the aberrant prion is much more resistant to normal sterilisation processes than other infectious agents such as bacteria or viruses (Bellinger-Kawahara *et al.* 1987a,b). Furthermore, the long incubation period of the disease before the appearance of symptoms, coupled with the absence of an *in vivo* test for the presence of infection, has made it very difficult to predict the progress of the disease in individuals and populations, both animal and human. Research has been unable to demonstrate the presence of aberrant prions in milk or muscle of known infected animals, though recent studies in mice suggest that muscle tissue may not be immune from infection (Bosque *et al.* 2002).

Much research has been devoted to understanding the mode of transmission of the disease, and this has focused on the recycling of infected material through the use of MBM in animal rations. While other hypotheses such as accidental cross-contamination of non-MBM feed, environmental contamination and vertical transmission from mother to offspring are still being investigated, the cumulative evidence to date points to MBM as the transmission agent (SSC 2001).

Two principal questions arise – What was the primary source of the first contamination of the UK MBM supply? Did changes in rendering processes in the 1970s permit the survival of prions that had been destroyed in the earlier process? Both questions have unsatisfactory, inconclusive answers.

The origin of the BSE prion is not known though many hypotheses have been suggested. These include suggestions that the BSE prion originated from a mutant form of scrapie protein, a natural TSE in *bovidae* or *felidae* or other wild animals such as African ungulates whose carcasses were rendered into MBM, a sporadic form of TSE, or a spontaneous mutation of normal bovine prion protein into an infectious TSE protein (SSC 2001, Horn *et al.*, 2001).

Whether changes in the rendering industry permitted the survival of prions is also unclear, though survival may be related to the cessation of the hydrocarbon solvent extraction of fat from MBM in the 1970s and 1980s (Wilesmith *et al.* 1991). It has been demonstrated, however, that aberrant prions can survive the batch processing and solvent extraction procedures that were in use before the change (Taylor, 1999).

5 Containment Measures

As the number of cases of BSE began to rise, various measures designed to contain the epidemic and to protect the human population were introduced. Throughout Europe, the broad nature of the responses has been:

- *Control of animal movement,* primarily a ban on exports of cattle and cattle products from the UK (1996) and Portugal (1998).
- *Elimination of Meat and Bone Meal (MBM) from animal feed.* MBM has been shown to be the principal agent through which BSE was transmitted between animals.
- *Removal of Specified Risk Material (SRM) from the food chain.* SRM (including spinal cord, brain etc.) from BSE infected animals is believed to carry a danger of infecting humans with vCJD.
- *Exclusion of older animals from the food chain.* Because of the ban on use of MBM in ruminants (Ireland 1990, UK 1994, EU 2000), animals born after these dates are presumed to be free of BSE (surveillance data generally support this).
- *Introduction of carcass testing for BSE.* Since January 2001, carcasses of animals older than 30 months (24 months in some countries) cannot enter the food chain unless they have been tested for BSE.
- *Improved disease reporting and surveillance.* This includes compulsory notification of BSE (1990), epidemio-surveillance of all animal TSEs (1998).
- *Improved control of animal feed manufacture.* This includes new regulations on treatment of MBM, increased sampling of feeds and restrictions on feed manufacturing licences to ensure exclusion of MBM.
- *Improved traceability of animals and animal products.* This includes universal standardised identification of cattle (and later sheep), creation of databases, compulsory labelling at point of sale identifying animal or animals of origin.
- *Classification of risk status of countries* to facilitate international trade.

All of these actions are included in EU legislation (**Table 1.2**).

Table 1.2 Chronology of principal EU legislation (European Commission).

March 1990	Compulsory notification of BSE
June 1994	Ban on use of proteins derived from mammalian tissues for feeding ruminants
March 1996	Total ban on dispatch of live cattle and all cattle products from the UK
July 1997	Prohibition of the use of SRM (mainly brain, eyes and spinal cord)
October 1997	Restrictions on trade in MBM
April 1998	Epidemio-survellance for all animal TSEs
November 1998	Total ban on dispatch of live cattle and cattle products from Portugal
July 1999	Lift of ban on dispatch of certain bovine products from the UK
December 2000	Temporary ban on use of MBM
December 2000	Extension on list of SRM (bovine intestines)
December 2000	Prohibition of the use of dead animals in the production of animal feed
March 2001	Extension of list of SRM (vertebral column)
July 2001	Lift of ban on dispatch of certain bovine products from Portugal

Source: http://europa.eu.int/comm/food/fs/bse/bse15_en.pdf.

1.6 Risk Assessment and Communication - the UK Experience

Much has been written about risk assessment (Kaplan & Garrick 1981, Hathaway 1993). Risk refers to exposure to danger. The first step in an analysis of risk therefore is to obtain the required knowledge about exposure so that a simplified formula can be proposed: Risk = danger x exposure.

Hazard identification and characterization are easily obtained when the problem has been previously and appropriately addressed *i.e.* when accurate detection tests are available (detection of a virus, a bacteria, a toxic compound). Exposure can be assessed through epidemiological studies aiming at observing the environment where the animals are raised and, for the zoonotic aspects, the connection with human beings. On the other hand risk assessment is difficult when the problem is not well defined, when the causative agent is unknown, when the problem occurs at a low frequency or when exposure is difficult to evaluate. Usually the lessons learnt from the past help investigate the future.

Previously recorded data sets are used as the basis for building prediction models. For many animal diseases, factors associated with an increased likelihood of an event occurring are still poorly defined or unknown. They only come to light through the study of naturally occurring cases. Risk assessment becomes a real challenge when the problem is completely new. The greatest difficulty is to predict events which have not yet ever occurred. In other words, how can the innumerable potential results of multiple types of wrong functioning of a complex connected process be evaluated? Mathematics helps, but numerous assumptions are required to make possible the calculations. On the other hand they oversimplify the equations and hence move away from reality.

The various responses to the UK BSE crisis have been examined by the BSE Inquiry Report (Phillips *et al.* 2000) and more recently by Jensen (2003). The inquiry found that although reasonable measures had been taken to address the potential risk to human health, these were not always timely or adequately implemented. Neither were they suitably communicated to the public. Government officials and scientific advisors have been criticised as operating within a culture of complacency and secrecy providing misleading representation of risk.

An initial assessment of the potential risks, addressed by the Southwood Working Party (Southwood 1989), was complicated by the uncertainty of transmissibility to humans and the further uncertainty over the mode, scale and consequence of the disease. This meant the indeterminate outcome of any precautionary measure, the effectiveness and costs of which could not be known.

Serving as a guide to action for the UK Government, the Southwood report concluded that the risk of transmission of BSE to humans was remote. This judgement however gave no indication of the magnitude of the risk or any reasoning behind it. In addition, no alternatives to the hypothesis that BSE would behave like scrapie were thoroughly examined

Given the difficulty of assessing the real risks and alternative theories, the report in its recommendations sought to gain public confidence. For example, based on the risk assessment, as a matter of 'extreme prudence' the report recommended a ban on the use of ruminant offal and thymus in baby food but considered the proposed labelling of products containing brain and spleen unjustified. The premises for these recommendations are not entirely clear, though it is possible that the observation that young animals were more susceptible to BSE infection than adult animals may have influenced the decision to protect infants. Nonetheless, the unclear premises led to confusion rather than confidence among consumers.

Despite the scientific recommendations of the Southwood report, under considerable external pressure from the parliamentary opposition, various lobby groups and the press, and rising internal uncertainty of the risks, a ban on the human consumption of offals (Specified Risk Material ban, 1989) was introduced. Representation of the ban to the public however clearly stressed the remoteness of the risk to human health, suggesting that the ban was a form of insurance rather than a necessity.

Public concern grew when two independent scientific studies demonstrated the transmissibility of BSE to cattle and to mice (Barlow & Middleton 1990, Chandler 1990) and when a scrapie-like spongiform encephalopathy was reported in a domestic cat (Aldhous 1990).

After the publication of the SWP Report (Southwood,1989) concern increased over the rising incidence of BSE and its possible difference to known strains of scrapie. An important premise for concluding the remote risk to human health appeared to be challenged. This however was never clearly communicated to the public or to those engaged with the enforcement of precautionary measures.

Later assessments of risk by the Chief Medical Officer and the Spongiform Encephalopathy Advisory Committee (SEAC) made further reassurances influenced by internal pressure. Though they considered potential for the risk to be serious, they suggested there was only a remote risk to human health, but, in contrast to the Southwood report, that this was only because the control measures that were by now in place were considered adequate to eliminate or reduce any risk to a negligible level (SEAC 1994).

When the probable link to human vCJD was announced in 1996, the credibility of scientific advisors and government officials plummeted. In retrospect, it seemed unlikely that there was enough scientific evidence at any time to consider the alternatives so small as to be declared remote. If such risks were remote it seemed unclear why some measures appeared reasonable to implement. That scientific uncertainties were judged to have fewer rather than more possible consequences was a major failure of the initial risk assessment.

The failure of the communication of risk during the UK BSE crisis was inherent in the lack of transparency of the scientific risk assessments. The scientific advice required the concise investigation of uncertainties and analysis of all possible alternative theories and hypotheses. All facts and interpretation of scientific advice must be communicated clearly and unambiguously in the public domain. The only way in which consumer trust will be restored is by ensuring that in future the highest levels of transparency prevail.

1.7 Meat and Bone Meal

The basics

During slaughter and processing 33 - 43% of live animal weight is removed and discarded as inedible waste. This material, which includes fat trim, meat, viscera, bone, blood and feathers is collected and processed by the rendering industry to produce high quality fats (tallow) and proteins (meat meals) that have traditionally been used in the animal feed and oleochemical industries around the world. Renderers in the EU process about 16 million tonnes, while those in North America process nearly 25 million tonnes of animal by-products each year. Argentina, Australia, Brazil and New Zealand collectively process another 10 million tonnes of animal by-products per year. Total value of finished rendered products worldwide is estimated to be between US $6 and $8 billion per year (Hamilton 2002).

Unprocessed animal by-products contain 60% or more water. When processing these raw materials heat is used to remove the moisture and facilitate fat separation. Globally, the rendering process reduces the total volume of animal by-product from 60 million tonnes of raw material to about 8 million tonnes of animal proteins and 8.2 million tonnes of rendered fats (Hamilton, 2002). Stored properly, these finished products are stable for long periods of time. Heat processing also sterilizes the product. The temperatures used (133°C - 145°C) are more than sufficient to kill bacteria, viruses and many other microorganisms. A recent study in the USA (Trout *et al.* 2001) showed that rendering eliminated *Clostridium*, *Listeria*, *Campylobacter* and *Salmonella* in raw tissues. Such high temperatures are also effective in killing the anthrax bacterium and destroying the foot-and-mouth virus. Unfortunately, it appears that rendering does not destroy the mutant prion thought to be responsible for Bovine Spongiform Encephalophathy (BSE). This has led to the ban on the use of animal meals in feeds in Europe and in many other countries, at least for ruminants.

The term 'meat meal' (which is used when collecting trade statistics by Eurostat and FAOSTAT) covers a range of products. It would be helpful in the present circumstances to separate the data into bovine, ovine, porcine and avian, as well as into meat meal, meat and bone meal (MBM), bone meal, blood meal, feather meal, etc. There can also be a wide variation between plants and batches in what goes into the MBM that is being prepared. If the ash content is high, this indicates that it contains a higher amount of bone and is referred to as MBM. If the ash content is lower it is referred to as meat meal.

Feed value

As a feed, MBM is an excellent source of supplementary protein, has a well-balanced amino acid profile and is high in lysine (usually the first limiting amino acid) (FAO 2002). In addition, MBM is an excellent source of calcium and phosphorous and some other minerals (K, Mg, Na etc.). The ash content of MBM normally ranges from 28 - 36%; calcium is 7 - 10% and phosphorous 4.5 - 6%. MBM, like other animal products, is a good source of vitamin B12.

In ruminants MBM can readily be used to replace most other supplemental protein sources. The protein is less degradable in the rumen. For this reason, it has been considered a good source of by-pass protein, suggested to increase milk production in dairy cows. Replacing soya bean meal or fishmeal with MBM gave similar performance results in pigs. Up to 10% replacement levels for soya bean meal in poultry diets showed no differences in gain and feed conversion and even higher levels were possible for turkeys. It was also successfully used in aquaculture feeds (FAO 2002).

MBM and extracted fat from slaughter offal thus represent highly valuable nutrients for use in the nutrition of non-ruminant farm animals and fish. For this application the appropriate sterilization treatment is an unalterable requirement.

In Europe, the MBM ban resulted in a need for alternative protein sources in feed. According to Abel *et al.* (2001), for all the protein from MBM to be replaced in the EU, about 2.3 million tonnes (MT) soya bean meal,

4.6 MT peas, 3.9 MT beans or 2.8 MT lupins would be needed (additional free amino acids not considered). Further, they note that plant meals are inferior to animal meals with regard to various components. Plant meals contain anti-nutritive factors which can negatively affect feed intake and/or nutrient availability. More accurate feeding of livestock (phase feeding) with adjusted dietary amino acid concentrations, however, would allow for proteins to remain at levels similar to that contributed by MBM. Thus in terms of ensuring amino acid supply, the ban is a minor problem. The differences in cost are also considered insignificant.

A further consequence of the ban is a reduction in phosphorous (P) supply which is not compensated by the use of plant meals. An additional demand for inorganic feed phosphates of more than 100,000 tonnes is needed in the EU (Abel, *et al.* 2001). At present, this is supplied by increased mining of rock phosphates. A general application of microbial phytase enzyme (which increases the availability of P from plant materials) in diets could partially solve this problem.

Disposal

The other part of the problem is the disposal of MBM if not used in feeds. The alternatives are incineration, co-incineration (cement industry, waste incineration or fertiliser processing), burial, landfill, biogas or composting. Most European countries are resorting to some form of incineration. However, this still implies initial rendering of the material and storage before incineration. Recent estimates by EFPRA (European Fat Processors and Renderers Association) give the incineration capacity in the EU as 2.5 million tonnes while the quantity to be incinerated is put at 3.6 million tonnes. Abel *et al.* (2001) also note the production of greenhouse and noxious gases produced by incineration. They calculate that combustion of 1 kg MBM causes about 1.4 kg CO_2, some further trace gases (NO_x, N_2O, SO_2) and CO. Of these N_2O (nitrous oxide) is the most dangerous because its global warming potential is 310 times that of CO_2 and because of its ozone depleting potential in the stratosphere. CO_2 dominates climate-relevant gas emissions from waste incineration, more than 100 times that of other gases such as N_2O (calculated as CO_2 equivalent). Real emission data of N_2O from plants co-incinerating MBM, are not known.

It has already been noted that high temperatures are essential for the sterilization of the material. Composting or other biological methods do not achieve the necessary heat to make the material microbiologically safe. Burial, landfill and even storage of dry material pose unacceptable environmental risks as they are subject to incursion of vermin, birds and other animals.

In any case, the costs of disposal are very high. The data of Abel *et al.* (2001) show that the total costs of the alternative use of 3.6 million tonnes of MBM varies from €1.0 - 1.8 billion. On average, every kg of MBM not used as a feedstuff incurs costs of about €0.32. This is nearly twice the 1999 supply price of MBM.

The future

A new Regulation (EU, 2002) laying down rules concerning animal by-products not intended for human consumption was adopted by the European Parliament and the Council in October 2002 and will apply on 1 May 2003. In particular, the regulation introduces stringent conditions throughout the food and feed chains requiring safe collection, transport, storage, handling, processing, uses and disposal of animal by-products. Under the

Regulation, only materials derived from animal declared fit for human consumption following veterinary inspection may be used for the production of feeds. The Regulation requires the exclusion of dead animals and other condemned materials from the feed chain, the complete separation during collection, transport, storage, handling and processing of animal waste not intended for animal feed or human food and the complete separation of plants dedicated to feed production from plants processing other animal waste destined for destruction. It also bans intra-species recycling and sets out clear rules on what can and must be done with the excluded animal materials, imposing a strict identification and traceability system, requiring certain products such as MBM and fats destined for destruction to be permanently marked to avoid possible fraud and risk of diversion of unauthorized products into food and feed. The control of movements of BSE Specified Risk Material (SRM) by a record keeping system and accompanying documents or health certificates is also required. The Regulation does not affect the current EU total ban on the feeding of meat and bone meal to farmed animals, which is a separate issue and remains in force without any date set to terminate it. However, the Regulation establishes clear safety rules for the production of meat and bone meal in case it is ever re-authorized for inclusion in feed for certain non-ruminant species, e.g. poultry and pigs.

The new Regulation requires the complete disposal, by incineration or landfill after appropriate heat treatment, of Category 1 materials (i.e., animal by-products presenting highest risk such as TSEs or scrapie). Category 2 materials (including animal by-products presenting a risk of contamination with other animal diseases) may be recycled for uses other than feed after appropriate treatment (e.g. biogas, composting, oleo-chemical products, etc). Finally, only category 3 materials (i.e., by-products derived from healthy animals slaughtered for human consumption) may be used in the production of feed following appropriate treatment in approved processing plants. With the adoption of this regulation, in the future, the environmental and economic repercussions will be reduced as only 2 million tonnes of material derived from animals unfit for human consumption (compared to the 16 million tonnes of animal by-products in case of a total ban) would need to be disposed of.

MBM could be used again in feed if appropriate legislation and controls are implemented. If SRMs are removed, fallen stock are excluded and the process ensures heat treatment at 133°C at 3 bar pressure for 20 minutes, it is assumed that the risk of infectivity of the BSE agent is reduced to virtually zero. Better classification and separation of different materials would ensure that non-infective supplies would be assured.

There is, however, a serious problem of public perception resulting from the publicity surrounding BSE. The feeding of meat meals is popularly seen as cannibalism. This perception will undoubtedly affect the acceptance of the use of meat meals in future and further exacerbate the problem of disposal.

References

Abel Hj, Rodehutscord M, Friedt W, Wenk C, Flachowsky G, Ahlgrimm H.-J., Johnke B., Kühl R. & Breves G. (2002). The ban of by-products from terrestrial animals in livestock feeding: consequences for feeding, plant production, and alternative disposal ways. *Proc. Soc. Nutr. Physiol.* 11.

Aldhous P. (1990). New fears on transmission. *Nature.* 345(6273): 280

Atkinson N. (2001). The Impact of BSE on the UK Economy. *MAFF UK Paper,* presented at IICA*; www.iica.org.ar/ BSE/14-%20Atkinson.html*

Barlow R.M. & Middleton D.J. (1990). Is BSE simply scrapie in cattle? *Vet. Rec.* 126:295.

Bellinger-Kawahara C., Cleaver J.E., Diener T.O. & Prusiner S.B. (1987a). Purified scrapie prions resist inactivation by UV irradiation. *J Virol.* 61(1):159-66.

Bellinger-Kawahara C., Diener T.O., McKinley M.P., Groth D.F., Smith D.R. & Prusiner S.B. (1987b). Purified scrapie prions resist inactivation by procedures that hydrolyze, modify, or shear nucleic acids. *Virology.* 160(1):271-4.

Bosque P.J., Ryou C., Telling G., Peretz D., Legname G., DeArmond S.J. & Prusiner S.B. (2002). Prions in skeletal muscle. *Proc Natl. Acad. Sci. U S A.* 99 (6): 3812-7.

Bruce M.E., Will R.G., Ironside J.W., McConnell I., Drummond D., Suttie A., McCardle L., Chree A., Hope J., Birkett C., Cousens S., Fraser H. & Bostock C.J. (1997). Transmissions to mice indicate that 'new variant' CJD is caused by the BSE agent. *Nature* 389(6650):498-501.

Chandler R.L. (1990). BSE scrapie and laboratory models. *Vet. Rec.* 126 (9): 223.

EAAP Publication no. 1/94. *LPS Special issue: Bovine spongiform Encephalopathy.* Elsevier, Amsterdam.

d'Aignaux J.N.H, Cousens S.N. & Smith P.G. (2001). Predictability of the UK Variant Creutzfeldt-Jakob Disease Epidemic. *Science* 294: 1729-1731.

EU. (2002). Regulation (EC) No 1774/2002 of the European Parliament and of the Council of 3 October 2002 laying down health rules concerning animal by-products not intended for human consumption Official Journal L 273, 10/10/2002.

FAO. (2002). *Animal Feed Resources Information System (AFRIS).* http:// www.fao.org/livestock/frg/afris/ default.htm

Ferguson N.M., Ghani A.C., Donnelly C.A., Hagenaars T.J. & Anderson R.M. (2002). Estimating the human health risk from possible BSE infection of the British sheep flock. *Nature.* 415:420-4.

Ghani A.C., Ferguson N.M., Donnelly C.A. & Anderson R.M. (2000). Predicted vCJD mortality in Great Britain. *Nature.* 406: 583-584

Hamilton C.R. (2002). Real and Perceived Issues Involving Animal Proteins. *Proceedings of an Expert Consultation on Alternative Protein Sources for the Animal Feed Industry.* FAO, Rome (In Press).

Hathaway, S.C. (1993). Risk assessment procedures used by the Codex Alimentarius Commission and it's subsidiary and advisory bodies. *Food Control* 4(4):189-201

Hill A.F., Desbruslais M., Joiner S., Sidle K.C., Gowland I., Collinge J., Doey L.J. & Lantos P. (1997). The same prion strain causes vCJD and BSE. *Nature* 389(6650): 448-50.

Horn G. , Bobrow M., Bruce M., Goedert M., Mclean A. & Webster J. (2001). *Review of the origin of BSE,* DEFRA, London. pp66.

Kaplan S. & Garrick B.J. (1981). On the quantitative definition of risk. *Risk Analysis*, 1, 11-27.

Jensen K.K. (2003). BSE in the UK: Why the Risk Communication Strategy Failed (Forthcoming in *Journal of Agricultural and Environmental Ethics*).

Phillips N. A., Bridgeman J. & Ferguson-Smith, M. (2000). *The BSE Inquiry: The inquiry into BSE and variant CJD in the United Kingdom,* Stationery Office, London; *www.bse.org.uk*

Politiek R.D. & Bakker J.J. (Eds.) (1982). *Livestock production in Europe. Perspectives and prospects.* Wageningen Scientific Publishing, Amsterdam, 335 pp.

POST, Parliamentary Office of Science & Technology. (2002). V-CJD in the Future. *Postnote,* Number 171

Prusiner S.B. (1986). Prions are novel infectious pathogens causing scrapie and Creutzfeldt-Jakob disease. *Bioessays.* 5(6):281-6.

Prusiner S.B. (1987). Prions and neurodegenerative diseases. *N. Engl. J. Med.* 317(25):1571-81.

Southwood R. (1989). *Report of the Working Party on Bovine Spongiform Encephalopathy,* Department of Health, Ministry of Agriculture, Fisheries and Food, UK

SEAC, Spongiform Encephalopathy Advisory Committee. (1994). *Transmissible Spongiform Encephalopathies: A Summary of Present Knowledge and Research.* HMSO, London.

SSC, Scientific Steering Committee. (2001). *Hypotheses on the origin and transmission of BSE.* Opinion of the Scientific Steering Committee Meeting, adopted 29-30 November 2001, EC Brussels.

Taylor D.M. (1999). Inactivation of prions by physical and chemical means. *Journal of Hospital Infection.*43, S69-S76.

Trout H.F., Schaeffer D., Kakoma I. & Pearl G. 2001. *Directors Digest* #312. Fats and Proteins Research Foundation.

Valleron A.J., Boelle P.Y., Will R & Cesbron J.Y. (2001). Estimation of Epidemic Size and Incubation Time Based on Age Characteristics of vCJD in the United Kingdom. *Science* 294: 1726-28

Wilesmith J.W., Wells G.A., Cranwell M.P. & Ryan J.B. (1988). Bovine spongiform encephalopathy: epidemiological studies. *Vet Rec.* 123(25): 638-44.

Wilesmith J.W., Ryan J.B. & Atkinson M.J. (1991). Bovine spongiform encephalopathy: epidemiological studies on the origin. *Vet Rec.* 128(9): 199-203.

Chapter 2. The Changing Context: an Industry in Transition

The BSE crisis occurred, first in the UK, and then throughout Europe, against a background of rapidly changing structures in the production, marketing and consumption of food. While these changes apply across the food and agriculture sector, they have been particularly marked in meat, and especially beef.

Some of these changes flow from the progressive liberalisation of trade within the European Union. A wider trade liberalisation under the World Trade Organisation (WTO) is also a factor. However, most change is a result of competitive pressures and technical and economical evolution in production, processing and distribution. Finally, changes in the nature of consumer demand have also had an impact.

It is beyond the scope of this report to provide a full analysis of these background factors. However, it is important to understand the impact of the main drivers of change. For many involved in production, processing or distribution, the constant adaptation to change made this an industry already in crisis, and ill placed to absorb the impact of a sudden new crisis such as BSE. Furthermore, the rapid change which has been taking place in the industry interacted with the BSE crisis, and in some ways contributed to it. Finally, the changes which can be observed in the industry will continue. In looking to the future, therefore, it is essential to understand the causes, nature, and probable consequences of structural change.

In that context, the following sections document the evolution of the food production industry in Europe and further afield.

2.1 The Changing Consumer

The patterns of production of food on farm, and of its processing and distribution are determined by the demands of consumers. A few generations ago in Europe, and still in many developing countries, a high proportion of consumers were also involved in food production. Consumer demand was very stable, and formed by traditional patterns of food availability. Today, food producers form less than 5% of the population and consumers have little connection with or knowledge of food production. In addition, with increased purchasing power and access to food from all over the world, consumers have no restraints on choice, and are subject to many influences which change the pattern of demand.

For those involved in the production chain, these factors create a demanding market requiring constant adaptation and new disciplines. The main elements affecting change in the market are as follows.

The total population of the EU15 is currently 379.4 million (January 2002). The total number of consumers in Europe has been increasing at a rate of about 2% - 3% per annum (2.6% 1999, 2.8% 2000) and is expected to reach a peak in 2023 returning to the current level by 2050 (Eurostat 2002). The total American market, as measured by gross expenditure on food, has been expanding at 1% per year, in line with population growth.

Consumers are becoming richer, and relative to other products food is becoming cheaper in the European Union. Gross domestic product (GDP) per head of population has been increasing at about 2% per annum (3.3% 2000, 1.6% 2001). The index of consumer food prices in the three years to 2001 was 104.4, 105.3 and 110.0 (base 100 = 1995) compared to the overall consumer price index of 107.8, 110.5 and 113.3 for the same three years. These trends combine to give a declining proportion of disposable income spent on food (**Figure 2.1**). In the EU15 this now averages 12%, and varies from 8.6% in the UK to 16.4% in Greece (Eurostat 2002).

In their food purchases, consumers are buying more services and less product. This is a result of complex changes in lifestyles, with time for food preparation becoming a steadily more important issue. It also reflects the increasing cost and complexity of food processing, packaging and promotion. One consequence is that the primary producer's share of the consumer's expenditure is declining steadily. This is most clearly demonstrable in the US market (**Figure 2.2**) where the producer share of the consumer dollar has declined from 33% in 1970 to 20% in 2000 (ERS, USDA).

A similar trend can be seen in Europe. Figures for the German market (**Figure 2.3**) show that from the mid 1970s to the mid 1990s, the producer's share of consumer expenditure on meat products fell from 52% to 30% and for dairy products it declined from 61% to 46%, in each case about a 1% drop per year.

Changes in the pattern of consumer demand are also driven by changing social structures: smaller families, more single households, working women, ageing population, urbanisation, foreign travel and many other factors. One major element of change is the increasing proportion of food purchased and consumed outside the home. Again, this has been documented in the US, where "out of home" purchases increased from 25% to over 40% between 1965 and 2000 (**Figure 2.4**).

Consumers are increasingly conscious of health and safety in food. One important aspect is the demand for lower fat foods,

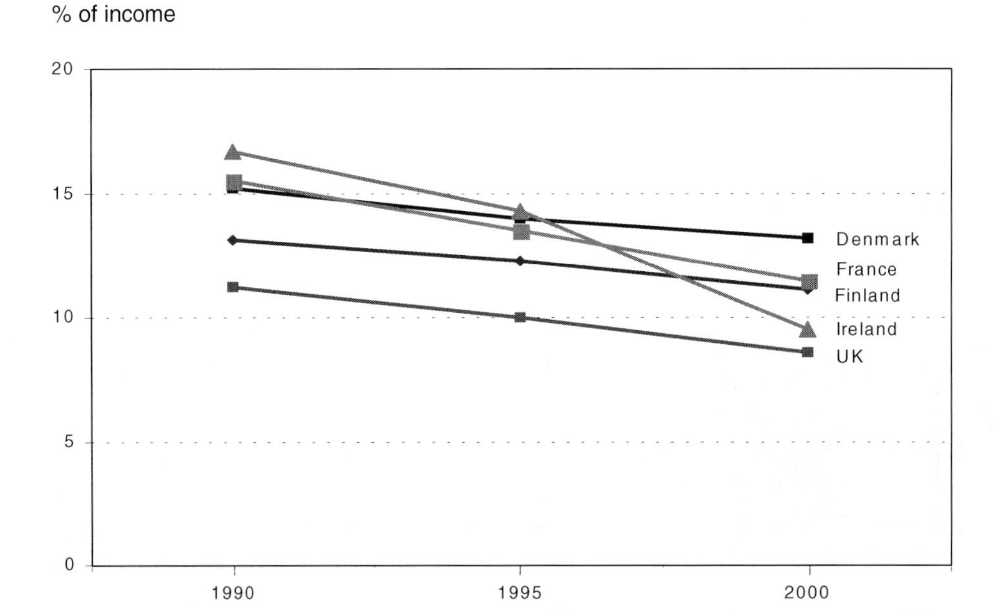

Figure 2.1 Food as percentage of disposable income. Figure includes all EU countries for which complete data were available (Source: Eurostat).

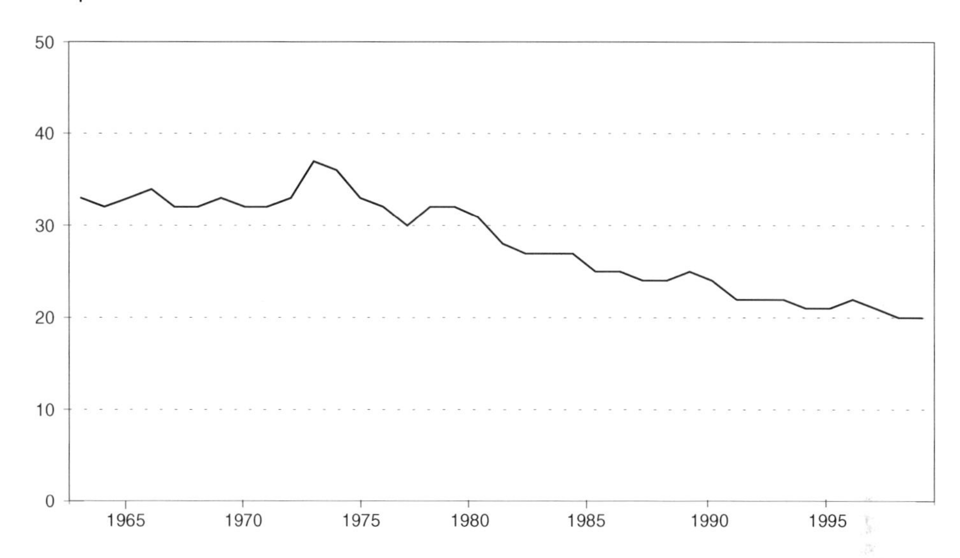

Figure 2.2. Percent of US consumer food expenditure going to farm producers (Source: ERS, USDA).

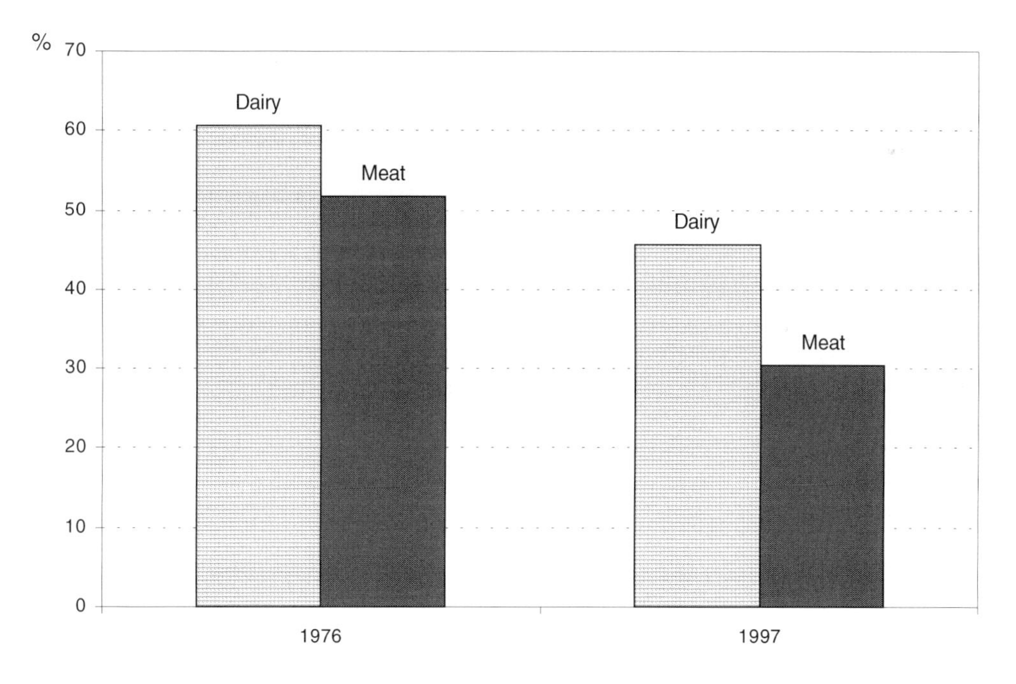

Figure 2.3. German producers' share of consumer expenditure for livestock based food products of domestic origin (Source: Weindlmaier, 2000).

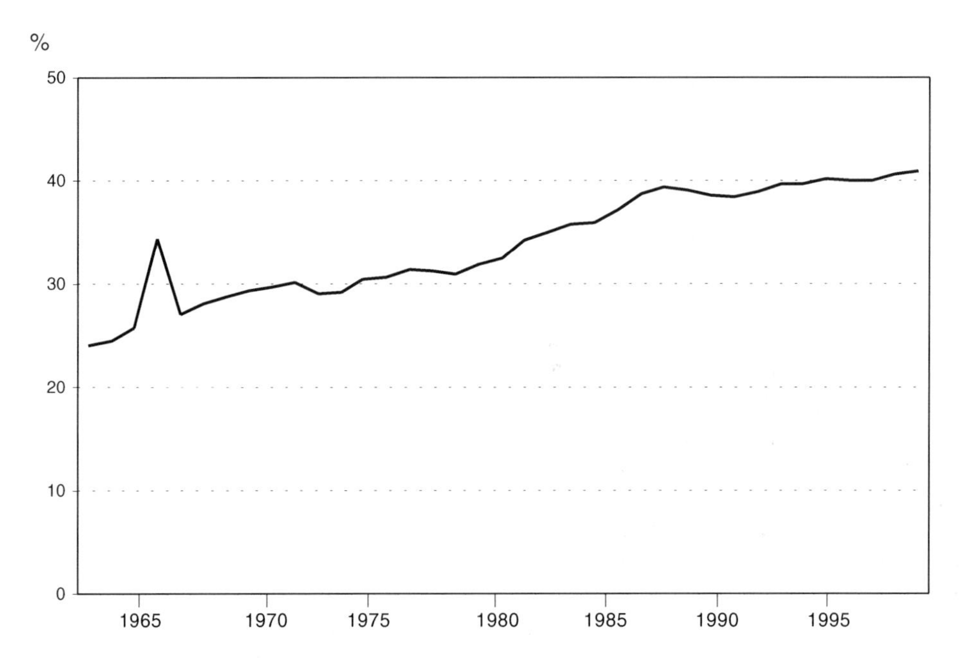

Figure 2.4. Percent of US consumer food expenditure for food "out of home" (Source: ERS, USDA).

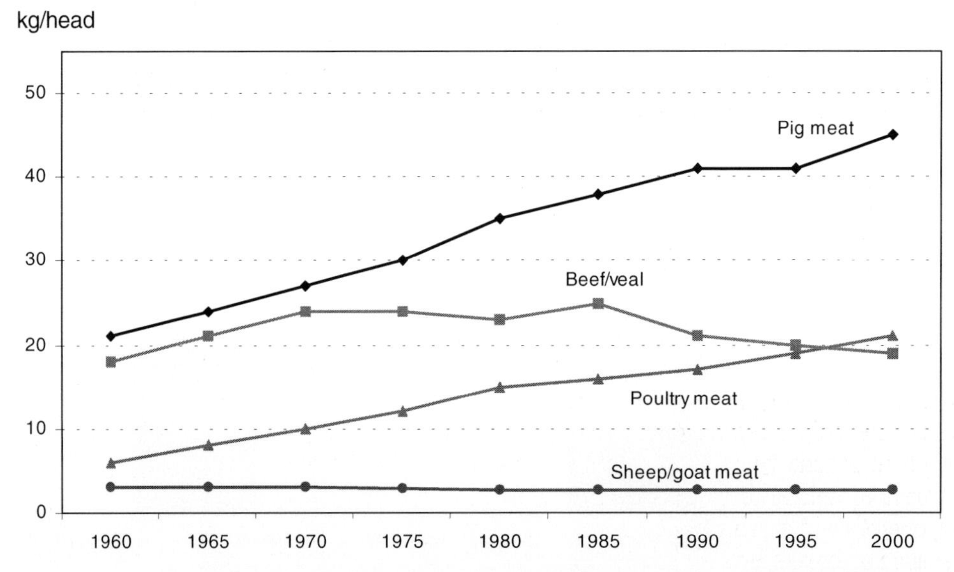

Figure 2.5. Consumption (kg carcass equivalent/head) of meat in EU 15 (Source: European Commission Directorate General for Agriculture).

which has had a marked impact on meat and dairy sales, and on preferences in the meat market. Another is the impact of recurrent crises such as BSE, salmonella, *E. coli* and dioxin on consumer confidence. One consequence has been an increasing demand for food labelled as "organic". Organic foods account for 1-2% of retail sales in both the EU and US. Expected annual growth in sales is about 20% in both markets (see section 3.9).

The consumption of meat in Europe has increased substantially since the 1960s, almost twice as much meat being consumed now (88.1 kg/head) as in 1960 (48.2 kg/head). Of particular concern to European livestock producers has been the shift in consumer demand between the four main meats. Driven mainly by price, but also by health, food scares and lifestyle issues, the per capita consumption of the main meats has changed steadily, and continues to change (OECD, **Figure 2.5**).

While overall meat consumption has increased, most of this has been due to growth in pigmeat and poultry. Beef and veal consumption per head increased from 18.2 kg/head in 1960 to almost 25 kg/head in 1985, and has since declined again to 19.3 kg/head in 2000. Red meats (beef/veal/sheepmeat) make up 26.2% of total consumption today, as against 45.4% in 1960.

2.2 The Effect of Food Scares

The largest and most economically damaging events affecting livestock production in Europe in recent years have been major outbreaks of animal disease, such as FMD, BSE, or classical swine fever. Apart from BSE, most such outbreaks have no implications for human health. However, they cause great economic disruption and loss, and have a significant impact on consumer confidence in the safety and integrity of the production chain.

In addition to livestock disease, there has been an increasing level of reporting of other food scares affecting the safety and acceptability of livestock products. Most of these concern the discovery of banned or unacceptable components in livestock feeds, or in livestock products. While it can be argued that the safety levels of livestock products have never been greater, there are a number of reasons why the level of reported food scares is increasing. The first is that such events are more newsworthy now than in the past. Secondly, the range of prohibited substances has steadily increased, providing greater scope for breaches of the law. Thirdly, levels of surveillance and analysis have also increased, both at official level and as part of the monitoring and control of commercial supply chains.

Though it is difficult to document, it is also possible that as intra community trade was facilitated by the Single European Act of 1990, the cross border flows of feed ingredients, waste materials and animals has increased the risk of contamination in the food chain. Three events illustrate this. The first is the rapid spread of FMD through a calf entrepot in France, from its origins in the UK, through Ireland to France and the Netherlands. A second is the recent discovery of MPA, an illegal hormone, in pig feed used on farms in 11 EU countries. Its origin was traced to waste material recovered from a pharmaceutical plant in Ireland, and marketed as a feed component by a company in Belgium. A third is the international spread of BSE through trade in meat and bone meal.

Some significant food scares affecting the European livestock industry in the first half of 2002 are listed in **Box 2**. These represent a small proportion of such events which are reported in the media. They also reinforce the memory of events such as the discovery of

Box 2. Food Scares in Europe, Jan-July 2002

January **Polychlorinate biphenyls in pig and chicken feed**
The Belgian Food Safety Authority (AFSCA) found traces of polychlorinate biphenyls (PCBs) in pig and chicken feed. PCBs, which were once used in industry, have been linked to cancer and birth defects.

February **Sulphonamide in chicken feed**
The Belgian Food Safety Authority (AFSCA) found traces of sulphonimide, an antibiotic that can contaminate eggs and cause skin allergies in humans, in chicken feed. Sulphonamide is authorised as a component of feed for pigs and broiler poultry but is banned in feed for laying hens.

March/July **Nitrofuran and Chloramphenicol in chicken**
The banned antibiotics nitrofuran and chloramphenicol were found in chicken imported to Europe from Thailand.

May **Nitrofen in chicken**
In Germany, wheat used in organic animal feed was found to contain more than 600 times the lawful level of the herbicide nitrofen. Traces were found in some organic animal products such as eggs, chicken, milk and meats. Nitrofen, has been banned in the EU since 1988 because it is believed to cause cancer.

June **Beef and pork protein in chicken**
Traces of beef and pork protein were found in chicken breasts imported from Thailand and Brazil and processed in the Netherlands. The added proteins allow the chicken to absorb extra water in a process called "tumbling" resulting in greater weight and volume of the product.

July **Hormones in pig feed**
MPA (medroxyprogesterone-acetate) a growth hormone banned in the EU was found in pig feed in 11 countries. MPA is a component of human hormone replacement therapies and may cause infertility. The source of MPA was traced to reprocessed waste from a pharmaceutical plant in Ireland.

human and animal waste used in animal feed (France, August 1999) and the discovery of dioxins in animal feed arising from the use of contaminated fats (Belgium, May 1999).

Such food scares are often compounded by evidence of fraudulent practice. This is well illustrated by the experience of Japan in the early part of 2002. Following the first case of BSE in that country in September 2001, and the subsequent collapse of the internal beef market, the Government introduced subsidies for domestic producers. In January 2002, imported beef was found to be re-labelled as Japanese in order to avail of these subsidies. Further investigation showed that low grade beef was labelled as high valued Wagyu product, and that similar practices had been in place in pork retailing, as well as in the presentation of imported chicken under a top Japanese brand name with false declarations on the labelling. These combinations of breaches of security, evidence of fraud, and constant exposure in the media have created a collective and pervasive distrust among consumers. The economic consequences have been huge, including the collapse of 64 companies in Japan.

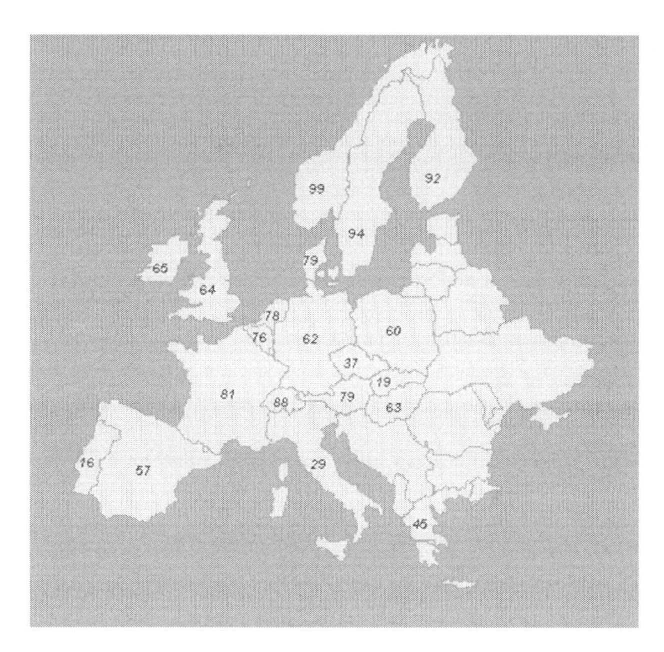

Figure 2.6. Food retailing: market share of 5 largest retailers in different countries, 2000 (Source: www.mm-eurodata.de).

2.3 Retailing and Processing: Rapidly Increasing Concentration

Up to the 1940s, food retailing in Europe was almost exclusively a local matter. Consumers purchased their food on a daily basis from small, family owned stores. Apart from a few internationally traded commodities (e.g. coffee, sugar) most items of food were produced within a few kilometres from the retailer. This was particularly true of perishable goods, such as milk, meat and bread.

In the post war period, the expansion of food retailing chains began. In some cases, these grew from existing producer or consumer co-operative enterprises, while in other cases they were based on the expansion of existing multiple store groups. The dominance of supermarket chains in food retailing has now progressed to a very high degree in Europe. Competitive pressures have meant that successful chains are driven to seek an ever-increasing market share. This has resulted in the dominance of relatively few chains in each market, and a growing dominance of the strongest of these across markets.

The present position in Europe is shown in **Figure 2.6.** In many European countries the top five chains have at least two-thirds of the food retail market. This dominance is highest in northern and western Europe, rising to over 90% in the Scandinavian markets.

As the barriers to trade within the European Union have come down, the largest food retailing chains have increased their market share across national boundaries. In 1990, the five largest chains at the European level held 13.8% of the total market, while in 2000 they had almost doubled that market share to 26.4%.

A similar pattern of consolidation and structural change is taking place in US food retailing, with the top 20 retailers having over

50% of the market, and the top four increasing their market share from 16% in 1992 to 29% in 1998. (ERS, USDA)

It is clear that this consolidation has potential benefits for the consumer in terms of price, choice and quality control. For producers and processors, there are both challenges and opportunities. One consequence of consolidation at the retailing end is that large retailers wish to deal with large suppliers. This reinforces the drive to consolidation in meat slaughter and processing. The trend is well illustrated in the US, where the four largest beef packing companies increased their share of all animals processed from 35.7% in 1980 to 71.6% in 1990 and 81.5% in 2000. (USDA 2002a)

The growth of these large packing firms in turn helps to drive consolidation at the production end. In the US, 45 feedlots of 50,000 or greater capacity provided 21.5% of all cattle marketed in 1996, while in 2000 the number of such feedlots had grown to 52 and their share of cattle marketed had grown to 24.5%.

These figures document a general evolution in retailing, processing and production towards ever larger dominance by very large scale enterprises. The pace of consolidation in retailing is as high in Europe as in the US, though in processing and production structures it is less rapid.

2.4 The Producers

There are almost seven million farms in Europe (2001) with an average farm size of 18.4 hectares. Approximately half of EU agricultural land is used for livestock farming. In Europe, animal output as a percentage of final agricultural output was 60% in 1997 compared to 46% in the US (OECD). In several EU countries, animal production exceeds crop production, the most extreme case being Ireland, where the livestock sector accounts for 90% of total agricultural production (Eurostat).

In the earliest stages of development, agriculture constitutes practically the whole of the economy. As economies evolve,

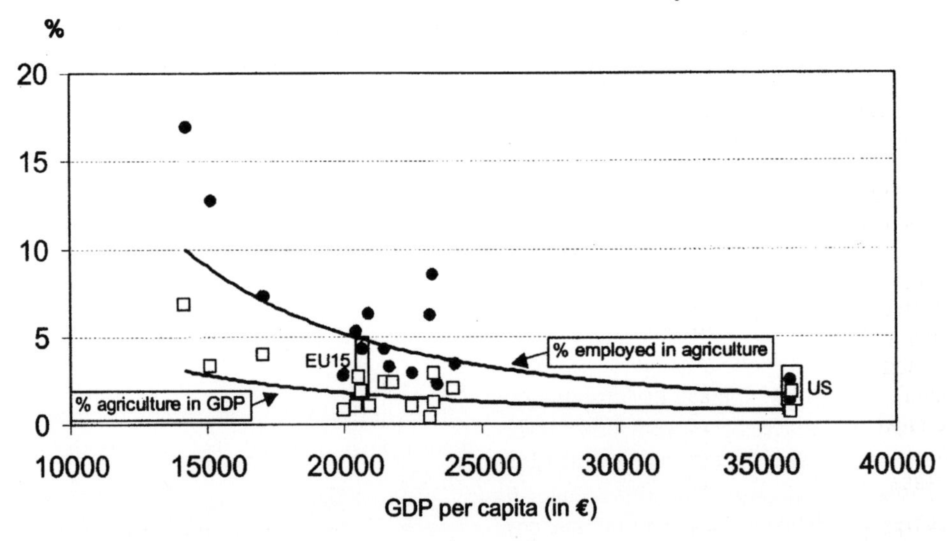

Figure 2.7. Agriculture as percent of GDP (□) and employment (●) in 15 EU states and in USA (Source: Agriculture in the European Union - Statistical and economic information, EUROSTAT).

agriculture continues to play a fundamental role, since food security is the first requirement of an ordered society. The place of agriculture can be tracked by two main indicators: the proportion of GDP generated by that sector, and the proportion of total employment that it accounts for.

The national economies of western Europe are among the most evolved in the world. The place of agriculture in these economies, as well as in the EU15 as a whole and in the US is shown in **Figure 2.7**. It is evident that as the wealth of society increases, the proportion of GDP accounted for by agriculture declines towards a value of about 1%. In general, the proportion of employment in agriculture remains at a higher level. In the EU15, agriculture accounts for 1.8% of GDP and 4.5% of employment.

With increasing GDP per head, these two percentages tend to converge. This general pattern illustrates the nature of the continuing adjustment in European agriculture, in which the largest element is the progressive reduction in employment on farms. This is recognised and facilitated by the Common Agricultural Policy of the European Union. Through a variety of mechanisms, this policy aims to support those on low income, while at the same time promoting improvements in the scale and efficiency of production units.

As is evident from the small scale of most farm units in Europe, many farmers cannot find full-time employment in their own enterprises. Figures solely for the livestock sector are not available, but a recent study documents the extent of part and full-time employment on farms throughout the European Union (Frawley & Phelan 2002). Eurostat figures for 1995 are given in **Table 2.1**.

Table 2.1 Employment status of farmers[1] in EU member states, (1995).

	Farming[2] (full-time) %	Farming[3] (Underemployed) %	Off-farm job[4] (Subsidiary occupation) %	Off-farm job[5] (Main occupation) %
Belgium	60	25	3	12
Netherlands	60	16	14	10
Ireland	52	15	25	8
U.K.	49	23	9	19
Denmark	47	22	11	20
Luxembourg	47	32	7	14
France	45	30	10	15
Germany	37	18	7	38
Finland	33	16	27	24
Austria	30	31	13	26
Sweden	24	22	20	34
Spain	23	49	4	24
Portugal	18	49	5	28
Italy	14	61	2	23
Greece	12	62	3	23
EU-15	24	48	5	23

[1]Person responsible for the current, day-to-day management of the farm;
[2]Farm operator (FO) has no other occupation and devotes 100% of a full-time worker to the farm;
[3] FO has no other occupation but devotes less than 100% of a full-time worker to farm;
[4]FO has an off-farm job but also devotes between 50% to 100% of a full-time worker to the farm;
[5]FO has an off-farm job but devotes from zero to 50% of a full-time worker to the farm. *(Source: Eurostat).*

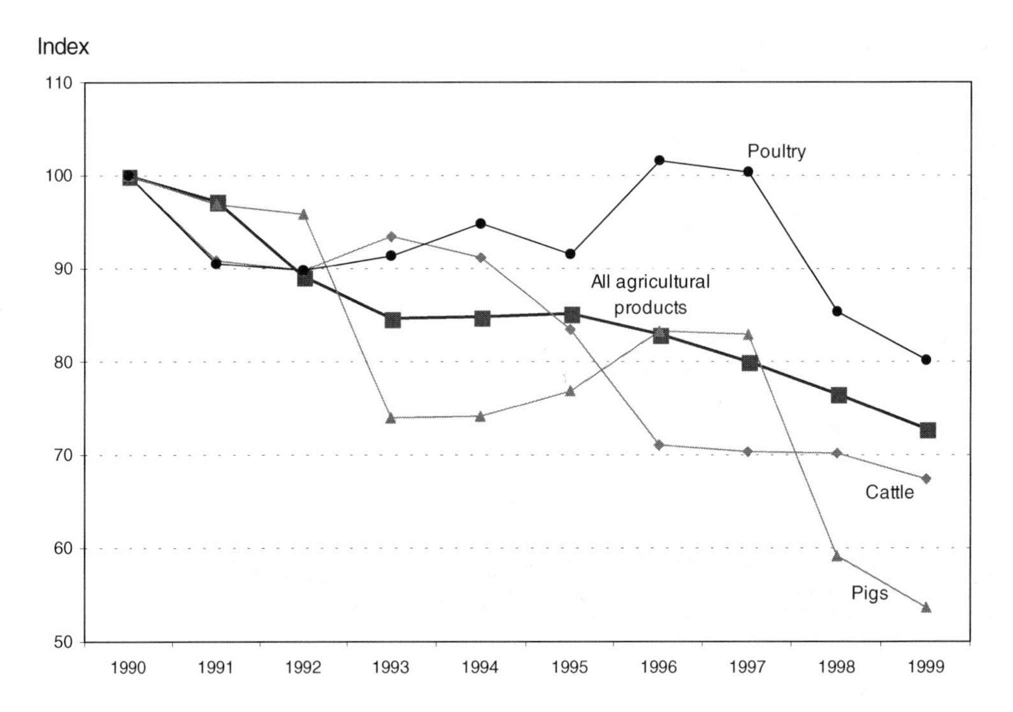

Figure 2.8 EU deflated index of producer prices (Source: Eurostat).

Less than one quarter (24%) of farms provide one full-time employment opportunity. Nearly half (48%) have no other occupation than farming, but are under-employed in the sense of having less than one full-time employment position on the farm. Twenty-eight percent have a significant off-farm job.

Behind these figures, there is considerable variation between countries. With some exceptions (Sweden, Finland), full-time farming predominates in Northern Europe. In contrast, it is generally less prevalent (under 20%) in Mediterranean countries.

This pattern of a mixture of full and part-time farming has a parallel in the US. There, the two million farm units are classified into small family farms (90%), large family farms (8%) and corporate farms (2%). Average farm size is ten times larger than in Europe. Over 50% are classified as livestock producers. Some 55% of farm operators had off-farm work, nearly two-thirds of these working in excess of 200 days off-farm (Hoppe *et al.* 2001).

The main factor driving structural change in farming is the low incomes of so many farmers. This is partly due to the uneconomic scale of many enterprises. It is also affected by the steady decline in real prices received by producers. **Figure 2.8** shows the experience of EU farmers in the decade following 1990. Agricultural prices generally declined at 3% per year with two major livestock products (cattle and pigs) suffering even greater rates of price reduction.

2.5 Scale and Intensification

As European livestock farming has changed, three parallel trends are evident:

Box 3. Bretagne, a Region of Intensive Livestock Production

The case of Bretagne is of particular interest (Mahé 2000). Despite the fact that the region covers 5% of French land, it produces more than 50% of national pork and poultry output, 40% of eggs and 20% of milk. Animal production represents 86% of the value of Breton agricultural output. Specialised pig and poultry production make up 50% of regional agricultural production. Together with the Netherlands, therefore, it is perhaps the highest density livestock economy in Europe.

The "Breton Model" has for a long time been considered a success in France, not only for its technical and economic efficiency, but also because it supported a very large number of viable farm units. These in turn are embedded in a network of small and medium sized companies, co-operatives and support organisations which provide an efficient range of financial, technical, market, transport and communications services. Because of its high dependence on pig and poultry production, which are largely unsubsidised enterprises, the region is less dependent than elsewhere on price support mechanisms.

In France, this model is now becoming less well regarded. Much of this changed perception has to do with environmental issues. For example, in Bretagne (1997) average nitrogen application was 228 kg per hectare, 60% above the average for France. Some 56% of nitrogen in Bretagne was organic, derived from manure spreading, as against 34% for France as a whole. Additional concerns for the public are emerging on perceptions of animal welfare in intensive production systems. Finally, there is a growing consciousness and resentment among urban consumers of the degree of subsidisation involved in agriculture generally.

These considerations are leading to pressures for change, reflected in the recent "Loi d'Orientation Agricole", which parallels the evolution of the CAP. In addition, commercial pressures in the same direction are beginning to be transmitted through to primary producers. The net effect is likely to be, at a minimum, stabilisation at present levels of intensity of production, and beyond that some degree of de-intensification. Paradoxically, this may lead to greater concentration of production, since smaller farms and businesses are more likely to cease production than larger ones.

Reference

Mahé, L.-P. (2000). L'avenir de l'agriculture bretonne. Continuité ou changement? Editions Apogée. 150 pp.

- Increase in scale
  - o Dairy herds, now averaging 30 cows (40% of herds have >50 cows), are increasing in size at 3% per annum.
  - o The average number of sows on pig farms has increased from 30 in 1987 to 43 in 1997.
- Increase in intensity
  - o Average milk yield per cow, in France, has doubled since 1970 to 6,000 litres.
  - o Growth rate and feed efficiency in swine have been improving steadily at 1% and 0.6% respectively per annum.
- Specialisation
  - o While this is difficult to quantify, most livestock producers now are committed to a single enterprise.

These trends are well illustrated by the example of Bretagne, a French region noted for the success of its livestock economy (**Box 3**).

Because these changes are interrelated, they are often confused. In particular, the effects of changes in scale and those of intensification in the use of resources are sometimes treated as if they were one factor.

A further source of confusion derives from the inclusion of all forms of livestock production in one set of discussions. Clearly, the land and forage based systems (sheep, beef and to some extent dairy production) require different treatment from those systems (pig, poultry, beef finishing, some dairy production) which convert bought-in feeds into livestock products.

One important form of intensification is the concentration of large numbers of livestock in small areas. This applies primarily to pig, poultry and beef finishing operations. Increases in scale are driven by the search for lower unit costs. Economies of scale for the operator, however, can often be more than offset by external costs, frequently borne by society. A recent study (Pretty *et al.* 2000) estimated that the "externalities" of British agriculture in 1996 were equal to 13% of gross farm returns and 89% of net farm income. About half of these external costs could be attributed to the livestock sector. It is clear therefore that spatial concentration of animals is an aspect of intensification which requires attention, and action, for the future.

For enterprises which are based on grazing or forage, the scope for intensification is limited by the carrying capacity of land and the seasonal pattern of growth. Thus dry Mediterranean grazing land may have a maximum capacity of 0.2 livestock units per hectare, and require seasonal movement of animals, while good quality grassland in the UK or Ireland may support 2.0 livestock units per hectare on a year round basis. The initiatives in EU policy (European Commission 2000) to promote extensification are directed primarily at reducing numbers of grazing livestock per hectare. They do not address the more environmentally costly problem of concentration of non-ruminant livestock,

The dairy industry is a special case. Throughout the EU, intensification, specialisation and increasing scale have proceeded in parallel. In the UK for instance, the average yield per cow in 1998 was 22% higher than in 1984, and average herd size in 2000 (73.3) was 9% larger than in 1995 (DEFRA). Through breed change and genetic selection, the cow population is highly specialised for milk production, and most dairy farms no longer have a secondary enterprise in beef or crop production.

Intensification in dairying has been achieved in two ways. Forage output per hectare has been raised to high levels (13 tonnes dry matter per hectare) by high inputs of fertiliser (250 kg N, 50 kg $P_2 0_5$). In addition, yield levels above 5000 kg per cow have generally been supported by purchased concentrate feed at a rate close to 1 kg feed per kg milk. With high stocking rates (2.0 livestock units per hectare) such systems can lead to progressive nutrient overloading of the environment.

2.6 Intensification and Animal Disease

The process of intensification of European livestock production has been underway for approximately 50 years. With the increased pressure on the physiology of the animal, and the progressive changes in its environment, it could be expected that parallel changes would be observed in disease prevalence and overall livestock health status. Widespread opinion holds that predisposing factors linked with intensification of livestock and farming systems are common to both the UK BSE epidemic and the more recent foot-and-mouth

Box 4. Cost of a Disease Outbreak - FMD in UK

The cost of disease outbreaks in the livestock sector can be very high. These costs are also very widely spread. Though livestock producers are the first to be affected, they may in fact not carry the principal economic impact. For many diseases there are publicly funded compensation schemes, so that taxpayers generally carry much of the cost. Secondly, the "collateral damage" to other sectors of the economy can be considerably larger than that carried by producers.

Estimation of the total cost of disease outbreaks, and its dispersion across the different sectors, can be difficult. However, the economic impact of the most recent large scale disease epidemic, FMD in the UK, 2001, has been carefully analysed (DEFRA/DCMS 2002). The outbreak began on a pig farm in the North of England in February 2001, and lasted for 221 days. During the course of the outbreak, over 6 million animals (0.8 million cattle, 4.9 million sheep, 0.4 million pigs) were slaughtered. Exports from the livestock sector (worth €2 billion in 2000) were largely suspended. There was widespread restriction of movement of animals and people throughout the country, with a major impact on the tourist sector. Some of these costs were immediate, while others will have an impact for some years into the future.

The total cost of the outbreak in the UK has been estimated at some €13 billion. This is more than the total value of UK livestock production in the year 2000 (€12 billion). Tourism and associated businesses carried the largest cost, amounting to €7.2 to €8.7 billion (low and high estimates). The public sector incurred a cost of €4.1 billion, farmers €0.6 billion, and the food industry about half of that. The economic impact on consumers was negligible.

Reference

DEFRA/DCMS. (2002). Economic Cost of Foot and Mouth Disease - a joint working paper by DEFRA/DCMS, March 2002

disease (FMD) epidemic. The costs of such breakdowns in animal health can be very great (see section 1.3 and **Box 4**).

Prior to intensification in Europe (<1960) the major animal health problems were both endemic and epidemic (Blancou 2000) and varied from one place and population to another. In cattle the main tasks of the veterinarian, besides individual interventions, concerned digestive disorders and parasites (internal and external). In many places tuberculosis was a major problem and had a direct relationship with human infection. In France, for instance, tuberculosis prevalence in bovine herds was approximately 25% in 1955 (Benet 1999). In pigs, diarrhoea, parasitism, erysipelas and peri-partum disorders were the main grounds for veterinary intervention. Where tuberculosis did occur in cattle, the infection could be transmitted to pigs by the feeding of unpasteurized milk and dairy by-products. In addition, faeces could also contain viable tubercle bacilli, a hazard where pigs and cattle are raised together which was often the case in European family farms at that time. Similar epidemiological links were found between avian tuberculosis and pigs (Biering-Sorensen, 1959).

Outbreaks of other notifiable diseases were also common. Rinderpest in cattle for example (Plowright 1965), despite having disappeared from western Europe by the end of the 19th century, occurred sporadically later (Belgium 1920, Italy 1949). Classical Swine Fever (CSF) and Foot-and-Mouth Disease (FMD) were also causes for major concern (Fuchs 1968, Henderson 1978).

In general, the first half of the 20th century in Europe saw farm animals faced with severe health concerns, several of which were zoonoses. This, and in particular the rinderpest epizootic in Europe, was the reason for the foundation of the OIE (Office International des Epizooties) in 1924, an inter-governmental organisation for animal health maintenance worldwide.

In the early decades of intensification in Europe, the efforts directed at genetic improvements led to large-scale animal movements sometimes over long distances without any serious concern for biosecurity. This resulted in the reoccurrence of epidemic viral diseases. For example, in cattle, Infectious Bovine Rhinotracheitis (IBR), already known in North America, spread massively in Europe. In pigs, Aujeszky's disease, a herpes virus first described in Hungary, also spread widely and Transmissible Gastro-Enteritis (TGE) (Goodwin and Jennings 1958) decimated thousands of young piglets during the 1960s and early 1970s. In addition to these "new" epidemics, "old" diseases such as CSF and FMD (UK 1967-68; France 1974) continued to pose problems, although now more sporadically as specific policies were adopted in different countries.

In the meantime, technical guidelines for intensive livestock production were progressively learned and implemented. Changes in herd management and husbandry combined with hygiene and prophylaxes (e.g. vaccination and de-worming) resulted in a profound modification of the overall animal health and disease scenario. Major zoonoses like tuberculosis and brucellosis were controlled. In France, the prevalence of tuberculosis in cattle came down to less than 5% in 1970 and 0.2% in 1990. It continues to steadily decrease. Likewise, health problems related to internal parasites like worms were solved. Other endemic diseases such as erysipelas in pigs nearly disappeared. Eradication plans were set-up and the major notifiable diseases like FMD, CSF and Aujeszky's disease became increasingly sporadic.

Whereas the situation improved regarding those well-defined (monofactorial) diseases, other disorders became progressively more prevalent, particularly those related to pathogen transfer through animal trading and inadequacy of on farm environmental conditions. Respiratory disorders for example increased in pigs, veal calves and beef cattle kept in confined housing systems and the occurrence of digestive disorders in pigs rose. It slowly became obvious that multifactorial diseases or syndromes with a quantitative expression develop on farms in cases of poor housing, feeding, hygiene and biosecurity. Only some of the technical elements of intensive livestock farming were known. In certain cases however, the knowledge was there but was not properly used, opening the field for endemic pathogen expression.

The current situation of livestock health in Europe can be summarized.

a) Major diseases that were formerly of primary importance (FMD, CSF, Aujeszky's disease) have been mostly eradicated. However, this does not mean total and permanent freedom. Sporadic outbreaks may occur locally if the related pathogens are introduced from infected areas. This was the case with FMD in the UK in 2001. The same cause can have the same consequences for other pathogens including parasites (Milne *et al.* 2001).

b) Major zoonoses (tuberculosis, brucellosis) have been eradicated though there may be possible sporadic recurrences.
c) Low impact of parasites especially internal parasites, which before intensification were a principal problem.
d) Pre-eminence of enzootic disorders relating to inadequate management conditions and shortcomings in hygiene maintenance. This does not mean that the conventional infectious diseases affecting livestock have totally disappeared. Influenza still affects pigs and other animal species, and Bovine Virus Diarrhoea (BVD) and Infectious Bovine Rhinotracheitis (IBR) still affect cattle. Control programmes are now being implemented. Conventional enzootic disorders were present prior to intensification but are becoming much more apparent and detectable in the current context.
e) Emergence of new and largely unpredictable problems such as BSE in cattle and Postweaning Multisystemic Wasting Syndrome (PMWS) in pigs.

Figure 2.9 illustrates the main trends in livestock health issues over time. The situation regarding disease is never fixed (Truyen *et al.* 1995). The mechanisms responsible for emerging or re-emerging diseases and the circumstances surrounding the occurrences are multiple.

2.7 Externalities

Intensification of livestock production and the integration of markets across countries have repercussions far beyond the farming community. The extent and magnitude of these changes have so far been incompletely

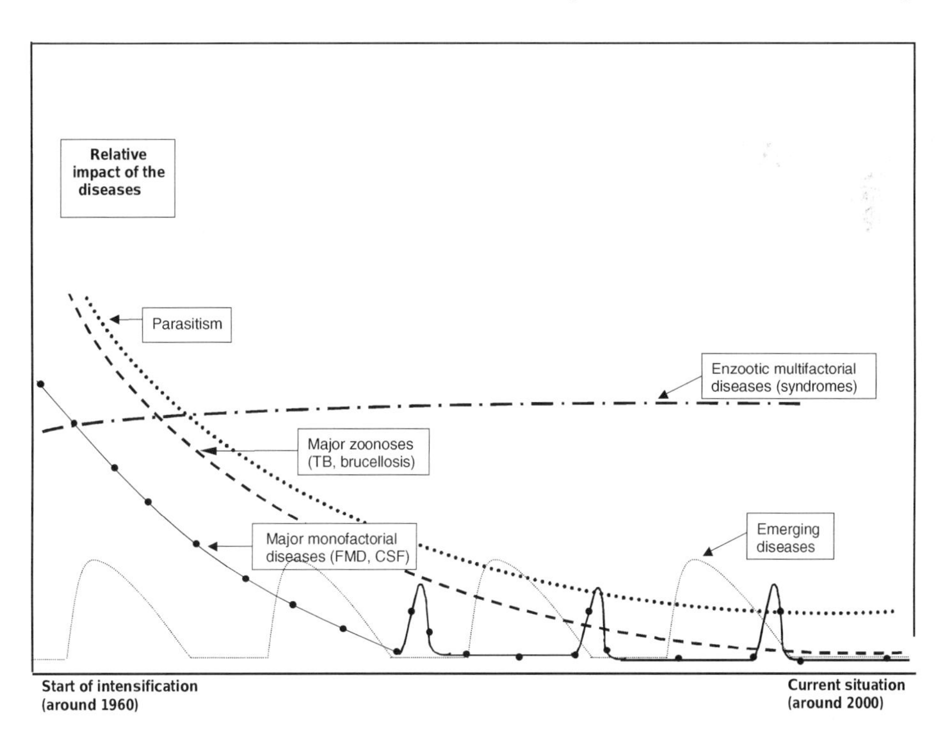

Figure 2.9. Schematic retrospective view of livestock health problems in Europe in relation to the intensification process.

assessed and only an indicative list of issues with partial estimates is available. The interconnections between crop and animal agriculture make it difficult to attribute externalities to one or the other sector for some of the identified issues. Further, the additional costs of intensification of agriculture that go beyond the costs of other forms of agriculture require quantification. These externalities, which need to be weighed against the benefits of intensification, encompass.

(Re-)emerging zoonoses

Intensive livestock rearing practices facilitate the (re)-emergence of zoonotic diseases by interfering with the ecological balance between microorganisms and their mammalian hosts. This interference can lead to changes in virulence, host spectrum and/or other characteristics of the disease agent. However, the impact of these re-emerging diseases has been dramatically reduced as a result of improved hygiene and animal husbandry practices. Overall, new diseases have been detected at a rate of one per year over the past thirty years. For example, the past decades have witnessed the emergence of enterohaemorrhagic *E. coli*, Nipah, and zoonotic avian flu.

BSE is the most notable and costly of the zoonoses that have emerged over the past decades. The emergence of BSE in the 1980s clearly shows how changes in production practices of agricultural inputs in conjunction with trading and feeding practices can alter the epidemiology and biological properties of a disease causing agent. Modern meat processing practices of the food industry have possibly facilitated the entry of the agent into the human food chain and in 1996 the disease was suspected in humans.

Food-borne hazards

Changes in food consumption habits (less meals prepared at home and more pre-prepared meals) coupled to changes in food production, processing (e.g. larger batches increasing the potential for and the effects of contamination) and distribution (longer distribution chains) have increased the exposure of humans to food-borne hazards. In the US, for example, food-borne diseases are estimated to cause approximately 76 million illnesses, 300,000 hospitalisations and 5,000 deaths each year, around 1,500 deaths being attributed to *Salmonella, Listeria* and *Toxoplasma* (Mead *et al.* 1999), pathogens of animal origin.

Compared to 1980 some countries in Europe have witnessed a 20-fold increase in the incidence of human salmonellosis, the majority of cases caused by *S. enteritidis* and *S. typhimurium.* In Germany an average of around 100 outbreaks of salmonellosis have been recorded each year since the early 1990s and the majority of food-borne disease outbreaks are linked to livestock products. A similar incidence of salmonellosis outbreaks is reported for the UK, poultry being the most commonly implicated foodstuff. The UK Food and Drink Federation for example estimates food-borne illnesses costing British economy around €1.6 billion per year.

Antibiotic resistance

Anti-microbials have been widely employed in the livestock sector, both for therapeutic purposes and for growth promotion, and a growing number of bacteria have developed resistance to a variety of anti-microbial compounds. Multi-drug resistant *S. typhimurium* emerged in cattle in 1988 in the UK and subsequently has been isolated from poultry, sheep, pigs and horses. It has stable resistance to ampicillin, chloramphenicol, streptomycin, sulfonamides, and tetracyclin. Infection with multi-drug resistant *S. typhimurium* has been associated with hospitalization rates that are twice that of other zoonotic food-borne salmonella infections and with ten times higher fatality rates. *E. coli* from animals are frequently anti-microbial resistant and transfer of that resistance to human organisms can occur. Antibiotic resistant enterohaemorrhagic *E. coli* O157 has been reported. Vancomycin resistance in enterococci associated with the animal use of avoparcin is well documented.

Some of these can cause disease in humans, which previously were easily controlled, but can now take a much more serious course. For example, a strain of *Salmonella* (*typhimurium* DT104), which is resistant to five different antibiotics has emerged and is responsible for an estimated 68,000 to 340,000 illnesses a year in the US alone (Glynn *et al.* 1998). Anti-microbial resistance in pathogens from farm animals can be passed on to bacteria of humans through the exchange of genetic material between microorganisms, thus increasing public health costs through the related use of more expensive drugs for treatment and longer hospital stays. For the US, the annual cost of anti-microbial resistance has been estimated to amount to some USD 30 billion (Institute of Medicine 1992). The problem of antibiotic resistance is compounded by the fact that no truly novel antibiotics have been developed over the last decade. While it is recognised that most anti-microbial resistance stems from inadequate use of these compounds in human medicine, evidence suggests that the use of anti-microbials in the livestock sector plays a contributing role.

The use of antibiotics in animals may increase the pressure towards drug resistance. However, by minimising drug use in intensive systems and a reconsideration of some farm practices regarding hygiene, housing and management in general could sustain intensive agricultural practices (**Box 5**). Research in analytic epidemiology (ecopathology) has to be promoted.

Animal disease outbreaks

In recent years the EU has suffered from severe epidemics of classical swine fever (CSF) and foot and mouth disease (FMD). Both are highly contagious diseases with major trade implications. Although disease spread can be curbed by vaccination, the use of vaccines restricts market access and stamping out is the conventional EU disease control policy.

In the case of CSF outbreaks in densely populated areas of the EU (in some areas there are up to 9,000 pig places per km^2), usually all pigs within a 1km radius of an affected farm will be culled (culling zone) and a total standstill of pigs will be imposed on an area with a 10km radius around an affected farm (surveillance zone). The standstill will only be lifted after laboratory confirmation that virus is not being transmitted any longer. Confirmation is obtained by serological examination of pigs not prior to 30 days after completion of disinfection of the last affected premises in the area. For areas with a high density of pig farms this may mean that thousands of pigs cannot be marketed for some time, yet require feeding and building space. Once the marketing ban is lifted, the pigs may have become too old to be profitably marketable and have to be destroyed. In the recent CSF outbreaks in the EU, around 8.8 million healthy pigs, i.e. the vast majority, were slaughtered under the market support programme for welfare reasons or because they had become too heavy to enter the market, not because they had contracted the disease.

Box 5. Reducing Antibiotic Use in Livestock Production.

For about fifty years, antimicrobial growth promoters (AGPs) have been used routinely in feed for healthy animals to improve growth rates and feed efficiency. Normally, they are incorporated in compound feed and do not require veterinary prescription. Many of the AGPs developed over the years are closely related to antibiotics used in human and veterinary medicine. In both of these fields there is growing concern about the emergence of antibiotic resistant pathogenic organisms. This is due to the natural selection pressure resulting from widespread use of antibiotics in medicine and agriculture. The contribution of routine use of antibiotics in livestock feeds to the overall problem of growing antibiotic resistance has been difficult to quantify (Isaacson and Torrence, 2002.).

Nevertheless, individual governments and the EU have moved to reduce antibiotic use in livestock production. In particular, the EU Commission in July 1999 banned the use of Virginiamycin, Tylosin, Spiramycin and Bacitracin, and in March 2002 proposed to phase out the remaining four AGPs by 2006. Prior to this, considerable advances had been made in the Scandinavian countries. In 1986, Sweden banned the use of AGPs in animal production. In 1998 use of AGPs was suspended in Danish poultry and pig production. This has led to a marked reduction in resistant bacteria from food animals (notably Enterococci, Ampylobacter and Staphlococci). There has been a parallel decrease in levels of resistance in bacteria from food (DANMAP, 2001). Studies from a number of European countries have shown a decrease in levels of resistance to AGPs in bacteria from the intestinal tract of healthy humans in the community (Emborg *et al.*, 2001), and there are preliminary indications of declining resistance in clinical infections.

The impact on the livestock sector is well illustrated by the Danish experience. While there was a temporary increase in the prophylactic use of some drugs, total usage levels in the livestock sector have been reduced by more than 50% between 1994 and 2000. The economic impact has been less than might have been expected. Broiler productivity and health has not been affected. Feed consumption has increased slightly (by 16 gm per kg broiler). However, the increased feed cost is more than offset by the saving from the elimination of AGPs (Klare *et al.*, 1999).

In pig production, average daily gains have continued to improve, and feed conversion rates have not deteriorated to any significant degree. There was some increase in diarrhoea in weaning pigs, but adjustments in management and feeding strategies are gradually resolving these problems.

It is clear that the intensive livestock sector in Europe cannot in the future use antibiotics routinely as it has in the past. The experience in Scandinavia and elsewhere demonstrates that with good husbandry these adjustments can be made while maintaining continued increase in the efficiency of production.

References

Isaacson R.E. & Torrence M.E. (Eds.). (2002). The Role of Antibiotics in Agriculture. A report from the American Academy of Microbiology, Washington DC http://www.asmusa.org.

DANMAP. (2001). Use of antimicrobial agents and occurrence of antimicrobial resistance in bacteria from food animals, food and humans in Denmark. A report from Statens Serum Institut, Danish Veterinary and Food Admininstration, Danish Medicines Agency, Danish Veterinary Institute.

Emborg H.D., Ersbøll A.K., Heuer O.E. & Wegener H.C. (2001). The effect of the withdrawal of antimicrobial growth promoters on the productivity in the Danish broiler production. Prev. Vet. Med. 50: 53-70.

Klare I., Badstubner D., Konstabel C., Bohme G., Claus H. & Witte W. (1999). Decreased incidence of VanA-type vancomycin-resistant enterococci isolated from poultry meat and from fecal samples of humans in the community after discontinuation of avoparcin usage in animal husbandry. Microb Drug Resist 5:45-52.

The cost of the market support programme amounted to €407 million and accounted for about 60% of the total control cost.

Foot and mouth disease was introduced into the UK at the beginning of 2001. The epidemic was brought under control within the year, but at cost of some €13 bn (see **Box 4**). Most of these costs fell on sectors outside of agriculture.

The reluctance by the authorities to abandon the rigorous slaughter policy, even after it had become clear that the disease was widely disseminated (subsidy-driven sheep movements are said to have contributed to its spread), was justified by the additional costs that would result from of an extended loss of access to export markets (gross worth of around GBP 0.5 billion a year) as a result of any disease control policy that would make use of vaccination.

Livestock epidemics

Trade facilitates the movement of animal diseases. Large numbers of susceptible livestock, kept at high stocking densities are extremely vulnerable to the introduction of highly contagious diseases such as FMD, CSF or Newcastle disease, demonstrated by the recent outbreaks of CSF in Germany and Holland and FMD in the UK and Argentina. Not only can diseases spread very rapidly in large animal populations and in areas with high animal densities, but also disease control measures in these instances often require mass slaughter of large numbers of non-infected animals. This puts a heavy burden not only on the farming community, but also on entire regions and countries.

Biodiversity loss

Domestic animal genetic diversity tends to be reduced by the trend towards the use of genetically uniform stock as scales of operations increase, as vertical integration of the industry strengthens, and as the share of conventional, diverse, small-scale production in the market shrinks.

Animal welfare

If not properly regulated, intensive large-scale animal production may be associated with management practices (e.g. space, light, movement limitations), which in some cases may not allow the expression of natural behavioural characteristics of the animals. Such practices associated with real and/or suggested animal suffering are increasingly resented by society. Similar reservations are also expressed with respect to animal transportation to markets and slaughter over large distances and to certain feeding and medication practices (Food Ethics Council 2001).

Pollution and nutrient loading

The main environmental problems likely to be associated with intensive systems are: 1) accumulation of animal waste, leading to build up of excess nutrients and heavy metals in the soil; 2) emission of ammonia and odours to the atmosphere; 3) emission of greenhouse gases: methane, nitrous oxide; 4) release of chemical inputs, feed additives and animal health inputs, tannery and slaughter house wastes; 5) degradation and depletion of fresh water resources and 6) high consumption of fossil energy leading to CO_2 emission and global warming.

The considerable volumes of waste produced by large-scale, high-density livestock operations can cause severe soil, water and air pollution. The most important emissions concern nitrogen, phosphorous, various heavy metals and greenhouse gases such as methane and nitrous oxide. Further, where recycling of manure and urine to agriculture is not firmly regulated, considerable environmental damage may arise.

Nutrient loading in crop-livestock systems may occur in areas where the nutrients present in manure are not properly recycled or treated. Even in well-managed systems substantial nutrient surpluses are normal (**Box 6**).

The major effects of animal waste mismanagement include eutrophication of surface water (deteriorating water quality, algae growth, damage to fish etc.) due to input of organic substances and nutrients; leaching of nitrate and possibly pathogens into ground water; and accumulation of nutrients, drug residues and heavy metals in the soil (Hamscher *et al.* 2000, Hooda *et al.* 2000, Schröder 2002).

The impact of livestock on nutrient fluxes in the European area has been estimated as part of a global study by the Food and Agriculture Organization of the United Nations. Statistics (1995 - 2000) on agricultural land, crops, mineral fertilizers and animal numbers (weighted according to species and production intensity to give total livestock biomass and total manure excretion) were used to estimate the phosphate balance at soil level per given agricultural land area.

The phosphate ($P_2 0_5$) balance, a robust indicator of livestock production impact on nutrient fluxes (Basnet *et al.* 2002, Gerber *et al.* 2002) is estimated as the difference between recognized inputs (manure spread and mineral fertilizers) and outputs (crop uptake) (Scoones & Toulmin 1998; Bindraban *et al.* 2000). Although spatial patterns and levels may vary, analyses of nitrogen balances demonstrate similar trends (Hoffmann *et al.* 2000; Hooda *et al.* 2000, OECD 2001).

Phosphate overloads can result in water system pollution in two ways: 1) by surface runoff, which threatens surface water and 2) by dissolved phosphorous leaching, which mainly concerns ground water. The most important factors influencing both diffusion modes are fertiliser application, land use, soil type and the Degree of Soil Saturation with Phosphorous (DSSP) (Hooda *et al.* 2000). In the Netherlands, a DSSP value of 25% is considered critical, above which significant phosphorous losses are expected to occur (Uunk 1991). By analysing nutrient balances, the speed at which the DSSP is progressing in the various regions of Europe can be estimated.

Nutrient loading throughout Europe is influenced by livestock density and the combination of manure and mineral fertiliser application. Mineral fertiliser applications, having risen steadily through the 1960s and 1970s, stabilised in the 1980s and have since fallen. Nitrogen applications were reduced following the introduction of the EU Nitrate Directive of 1991, which set a limit of 170 kg N/ha/year. Phosphorous applications in particular are now below the levels of 1960 (**Figure 2.10**). Throughout much of northern and central Europe, manure application is now responsible for over half of the $P_2 0_5$ supply in agricultural land (**Figure 2.11c**).

The broad pattern of nutrient loading of the environment follows closely the distribution of total livestock density (**Figure 2.11a**). Livestock densities can be divided into three categories:

High: High density areas (>500 kg biomass/ha) are characterized by high intensity dairying (>2 livestock units/forage ha plus >1.5 tonnes concentrate/cow) and high proportions of monogastric species (De

Box 6. Nitrogen and Phosphorous Flows in Danish Agriculture

While Denmark is not the most intensively used area in Europe for animal agriculture, it does have a high level of intensity of both crops and livestock, and an unusually high degree of integration between them. Land use is carefully regulated and monitored. One consequence of this careful management is that nutrient flows are exceptionally well documented (Kyllingsbaek, A., 2000, 2002).

The principal nutrients, and therefore the main potential pollutants, are nitrogen and phosphorous. Figure 1 shows the balance of input and offtake of these nutrients for both the crop and livestock sectors for the year 1998/1999. Both nutrients are in substantial surplus. Only 33% of the nitrogen input and 45% of the phosphorous input are accounted for by plant and animal offtake. For nitrogen, the surplus amounted to 153 kg per hectare, and for phosphorous 17 kg per hectare. These levels of annual surplus have come down substantially from the historically high levels of the 1980s, by about 15% in the case of nitrogen and 30% in the case of phosphorous. This reduction has been due mainly to reduced fertiliser use, though increased animal offtake has also contributed.

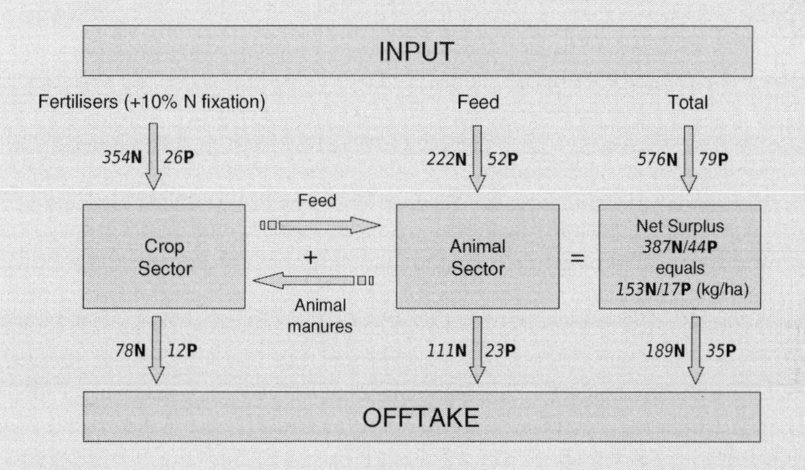

Nitrogen and Phosphorous flows in Danish Agriculture, 1998/99. Figures are '000 tons of N or P. Area used is 2.53 m.Ha (excludes set aside with grass) (Source: Kyllingsbaek, 2000, 2002).

References

Kyllingsbaek, A. (2000). Kvaelstofbalancer og kvaelstofoverskud i dansk landbrug 1979-1999. DJF rapport No. 36. Markbrug

Kyllingsbaek, A. (2002). Danish Inst. Agric. Sci. (personal communication)

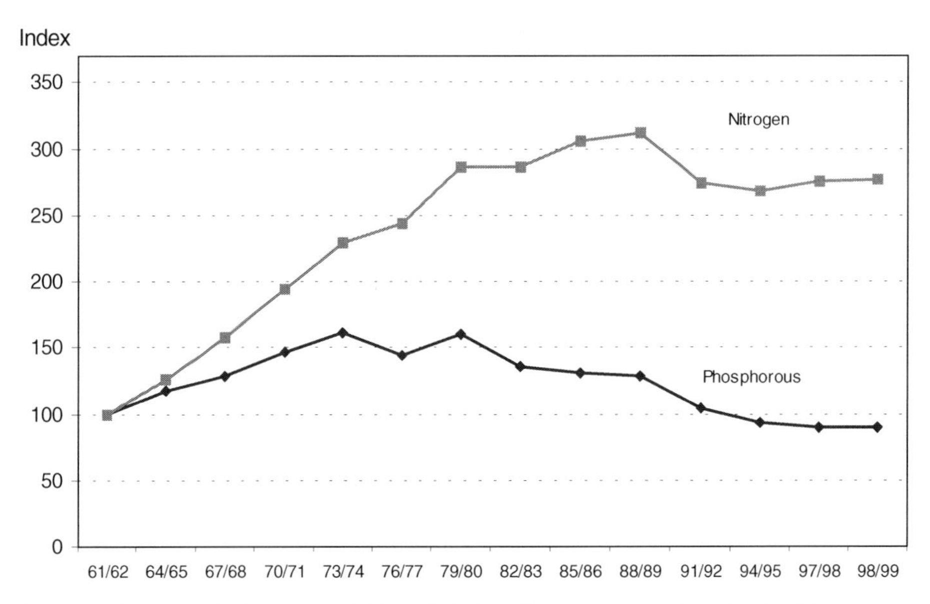

Figure 2.10. Trends in mineral N and P fertiliser consumption in 16 European countries (Source: International Fertiliser Industry Association 2000)

Haan *et al.* 1997). High phosphate overloads are generally evident in these areas (**Figure 2.11b**). The nutrient overload attributable to the contribution of manure to total P_2O_5 supply on agricultural land is shown in **Figure 2.11c**. When this is considered, areas with high livestock densities and substantial mineral fertilizer application (e.g. Netherlands, Brittany, Catalonia) have very high overloads (>70 kg/ha), whereas areas with high animal densities and low mineral fertilizer application (e.g. west UK, Denmark, northern Germany) have low (10-20 kg/ha) to moderate (20-40 kg/ha) overloads. Local surveys in the Netherlands have shown that a total area of 270,000 ha in the sandy areas of the central, eastern and southern regions are phosphate saturated due to intensive application of livestock wastes (Hooda *et al.* 2000).

Medium: Medium density areas (200-500 kg biomass/ha) are broadly suitable for forage production with lower intensity dairying, more beef and sheep production and monogastric species constituting less than 50 percent of the livestock mass. In these areas, the combination of manure and mineral fertilizer application is also critical to the nutrient balance situation. In Northern Italy and Ireland for example, the combination of medium animal densities and high mineral fertilizer applications results in high overloads (>40 kg/ha). Conversely, in central France, central Germany and Spain, balances are lower (<20 kg/ha).

Low: Low intensity areas (0-200 kg biomass/ha) are broadly in the Mediterranean zones of Greece, Southern Italy, France, Spain and Portugal, Scandinavian countries, and the specialized cereal zones of central France and Eastern England. In these areas little or no phosphate overload related to livestock production is evident.

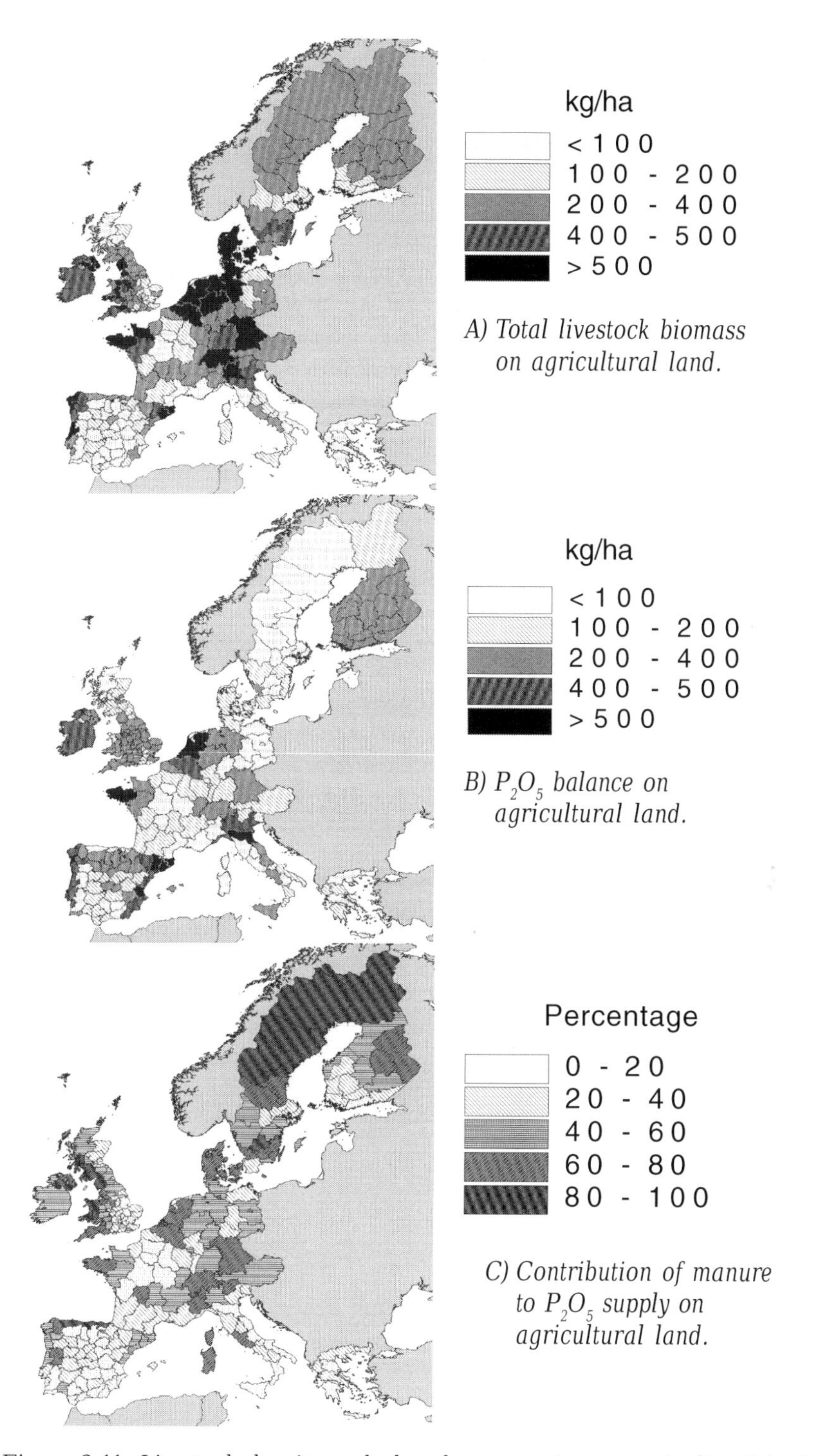

A) Total livestock biomass on agricultural land.

B) P_2O_5 balance on agricultural land.

C) Contribution of manure to P_2O_5 supply on agricultural land.

Figure 2.11. Livestock density and phosphorous status on agricultural land (Source FAO).

2.8 Trade and Competitiveness

Europe as a whole, including the EU15, is largely self sufficient for livestock products (**Table 2.2**). Nevertheless, because of the scale of the internal market (379 million consumers) it is the world's largest importer and exporter (e.g. 41% of world market in pigmeat) for several of these products. In 1998 the EU accounted for 14% - 31% of the total world exports of meat, butter, milk, and eggs. In addition, a substantial proportion of EU intensive livestock production depends on imported feed grains and protein sources (**Table 2.3**).

In the world as a whole, demand and supply of livestock products are rising faster than for non-livestock foods. Between 1987 and 1997 annual growth rates for milk and dairy products, meat and cereals were 0.3%, 1.8% and 1.4% respectively, and are projected to be 1.4%, 1.7% and 1.1% between 1995/97 and 2015 (FAO 2002). This demand is driven largely by expanding populations and rising incomes in developing countries where the annual demand growth rates for the above foods are 3.4% (milk), 5.9% (meat) and 2.5% (cereals). With this expanding market, international trade in livestock products and the raw materials used in their production is also expanding.

The future of the European livestock sector is therefore substantially involved with developments in international trade. In the past, trade policy in each country was determined at national level, in national interest. More often than not, this interest was seen as best served by a degree of protection

Table 2.2 Meat and milk production and self-sufficiency (1999) in the EU15.

	Production		
	Mt	%	Self-sufficiency %
Beef & Veal	7.8	21	101
Pigmeat	18.1	49	108
Poultrymeat	8.9	24	109
Sheep & Goat meat	1.1	3	81
Other meat	1.9	5	93
Total meat	36.8	100	105
Milk	126.5	100	108*

*Sources: European Commission 2000, Directorate-General for Agriculture, FAOSTAT and *Bundesministerium fur Verbrauchschutz, Ernahrung und Landwirtschaft, Bonn http://www.verbraucherministerium.de.*

Table 2.3 EU15 livestock feed requirements (Source: The Agricultural Situation in the European Union, 2000 Report, p. 85).

	Total (Mt)	Produced in EU	Imported
High protein	56	21	36
High energy	39	22	17
Cereals	110	108	2
Total	205	150	55

against outside competition. In other cases (as in the repeal of the UK Corn Laws in 1846) it was served by the trade liberalisation. In yet other instances it may be served by policies which promote or subsidise exports. Within the European Union, policy in these matters is now decided at EU level. Given the planned enlargement to include most countries of eastern Europe in the coming years, practically the whole of the continent will be covered by EU policy.

In its external relations, this policy is operated within the framework set by the World Trade Organisation (WTO). The broad objective of the WTO agreements is to promote ordered trade by the establishment of common trading rules and by the progressive removal of impediments to free trade.

Within this context, the greatest challenge faced by the European livestock sector is the long-term adaptation to competition from lower cost producers in other countries. In the short term, this competition comes mainly from the US and other developed economies with large land resources. Increasingly, there is also competition from developing economies such as Thailand and Brazil. In the future, there is likely to be an increase in competition from eastern Europe as the structural inefficiencies in Russian and Ukrainian agriculture are resolved.

Competition between the European livestock sector and those in other developed countries is affected first by the relative scale of production units (**Table 2.4**). Though farm sizes are steadily increasing, agricultural land per person in the EU is low compared with other major developed regions.

Since agricultural land in the EU is relatively limited, a more intensive pattern of land use has evolved. Farmers endeavour to maximise production per hectare by high levels of external inputs (**Table 2.5**). A further means of increasing farm income on limited space is by adding value to crops (grain) through livestock production; in addition, grain feeding removes seasonality of production and thus ensures a more even cash flow. The consequences are high livestock concentrations in the EU with concomitant animal health, welfare and environmental implications in intensive, often 'land-detached' production systems.

As a result of the high use of production inputs and of the 'value added' through livestock, gross value of production in the EU, measured per hectare, is very high, and, despite very low pasture availability, more than half of the gross value of agricultural production comes from the livestock sector. On the other hand, as land per agricultural production unit is low, gross

Table 2.4 Agricultural land per person, proportion of population in agriculture, area of permanent pasture and arable land per person in agriculture. (Source: FAOSTAT, 2000).

	Agricultural land / head of population (Ha)	Population in agriculture (%)	Permanent pasture (Ha/person in agriculture)	Arable land (Ha/person in agriculture)	Ratio Pasture/Arable
EU15	0.4	4.5	3	5	0.7
Canada	2.4	2.6	36	56	0.6
USA	1.5	2.3	38	28	1.3
Australia	24.3	4.7	466	55	8.4
New Zealand	4.3	8.9	39	10	4.1

value of production per person in agriculture in the EU is lower than in the US, Canada, Australia and New Zealand (**Table 2.6**).

Within the WTO structure, the most important relationship is that between the EU15 and the US. This is partly because they are the dominant trading blocks, and also because the positions which they agree effectively determine the WTO rules. Starting with the Uruguay Round Agreement on Agriculture (1994) agreement was reached on a range of measures aimed at converting variable import levies to tariffs, and progressively reducing all trade distorting export subsidies. Prior to this, the EU, under the first CAP reform adopted in 1992, had begun the process of shifting supports from prices to direct payments. The second CAP reform, Agenda 2000, continued that process with increasing emphasis on environmental aspects of production systems. In 2000, the net income of EU agricultural producers was made up as follows: 63% net returns from the market, 28% from subsidies on products and 8% from subsidies on production.

The net effect of all subsidies to agricultural production is calculated on a standard basis by OECD, and expressed in the form of Producer Support Estimate (PSE) percent. For the years 1986 - 1988, the average PSE in the EU was 44% (US 25%). For 1998 - 2000, the corresponding figures were: EU 40%, US 23%. In the EU this support system accounted for 1.3% of GDP and approximately half of

Table 2.5 Intensity of factor use (Source: FAOSTAT, 2000).

	Fertilizer T/1000 ha agricultural land	Tractors/ 1000 ha agricultural land	Harvesters/ 1000 ha arable land	Cattle/ 1000 ha pasture	Pigs/ 1000 ha arable land	Chickens/ 1000 ha arable land
EU15	121	49	7	1 445	1 667	13 421
Australia	5	1	1	66	55	1 907
Canada	35	10	3	445	272	3 402
New Zealand	40	5	2	674	237	8 167
USA	48	11	4	414	352	9 720

Table 2.6 Gross value of production per hectare and per person in agriculture (expressed in 'International $' of 1989-91) (Source: FAOSTAT, 2000).

	Gross value of production / ha agricultural land	Gross value of production / person in agriculture	Proportion from livestock (%)
EU15	1 245	10 352	53
Australia	51	26 315	58
Canada	317	28 946	42
New Zealand	421	20 391	91
USA	422	27 785	47

the total EU budget. Though subsidy levels as percent of output value are lower in the US, average payments to individual producers were four times as high as in the EU.

The 2002 US Farm Bill (USDA 2002b) provides for an increase of 70% in the support available to US agriculture for the coming decade. The 2002 mid-term review of the EU provides more for redistribution than for increases in total supports in Europe. In addition, the CAP must provide for enlargement and integration of the agricultural sector in Eastern European countries. The relative subsidy positions in future years are therefore difficult to predict. However, the US commitment to substantial increases in support in the medium term, coupled with the traditional position where 25% of US farm output went to export markets, seems likely to put long term downward pressure on world commodity prices. The net result for European producers could be greater difficulty, both financially and politically, in finding export markets for the smaller percentage of their production which is surplus to internal market requirements.

Competitiveness

The competitive positions of different economies are a reflection of the basic production costs of commodities. These are very difficult to establish in a comparative manner because of variable quality of data and differing conventions. However, a recent study (Boyle *et al.*, 2002) has produced estimates of comparative production costs for the main agricultural commodities across a range of European and other countries. A summary of the results is presented in **Table 2.7**.

The comparisons are made on the basis of 'cash' costs. These exclude structural features which also can have a bearing on competitiveness, e.g. exchange rates, indebtedness of producers, and whether land is owned or rented. They do, however, capture the main contributors to competitiveness: unit scale, climate, infrastructure, sophistication of services, and technical efficiencies.

As the authors acknowledge, in some commodities special factors may also affect the results. For example, in milk production, there is an apparent improvement in the competitive position of Europe and other areas relative to New Zealand. This, however, may be partly due to the costs of the rapid expansion in dairy production in New Zealand (58% over the decade considered). In addition, in the EU, increased milk quota values are not counted as a component of "cash" costs, giving an apparent advantage to the EU producer. In contrast to these results, other studies (e.g. Danish Cattle Federation, 2002) show EU milk production costs at 250% of those in New Zealand.

Table 2.7 shows results for four commodities: milk, beef, sheepmeat and wheat. The resources used in the first three commodities are largely tied to the local land base. For intensive pig and poultry production, feed constitutes 70 - 80% of production cost, and cereal production cost could therefore be taken as a surrogate for competitiveness in these industries. However, since cereals are a relatively freely traded commodity internationally, differences in raw material costs for pig and poultry production do not vary greatly between countries. Relative advantage in these industries is therefore more a consequence of other factors such as proximity to market, intensity of technology and scale of operation.

The figures show that for all four commodities, production costs in European countries are higher than elsewhere, and significantly higher than those of the lowest cost producer.

Table 2.7 Relative cash production costs per kg of product in different countries, 1988/89 and 1998/89. Lowest cost producer is given a value of 100. [a]1999/00, [b]1993/94. (Source: Boyle et al. 2002).

	1988/89	*1998/99*
	Milk: relative to NZ = 100	
Germany	286	118
France	229	118
Italy	286	106
Belgium	186	82
Netherlands	271	129
Denmark	371	159
Ireland	214	106
United Kingdom	243	124
Average	*261*	*118*
United States	329	159
Australia	114	76
Canada	243	165
New Zealand	100	100[a]
	Beef: relative to Argentina = 100	
Germany	355	328
France	345	317
Ireland	239	356
United Kingdom	329	439
Average	*317*	*360*
Australia	155	250
Argentina	100	100
	Wheat: relative to Canada = 100	
France	114	153
Denmark	229	237
Ireland	129	169
United Kingdom	186	186
Average	*164*	*186*
United States	100	92
Canada	100	100
Australia	86	129
	Sheep meat: relative to NZ = 100	
France	237	314
Ireland	171	327
United Kingdom	220	424
Average	*209*	*355*
New Zealand	100[b]	100

Productivity in the Livestock Sector

The record of improvement in technical efficiency in the livestock sector in the last half century has been remarkable. Fuglie *et al.* (2000) have documented changes in partial productivity measures for different sectors of livestock production in the US in the decades since 1955 (**Figure 2.12**). It can bee seen that, on these measures, pork productivity has doubled, milk output per cow trebled and productivity in beef and poultry production has increased by up to 50%. These figures translate into improvements in productivity ranging between 0.5% and 2.3% per annum sustained over a forty year period.

These gains in productivity have been the result of steady improvements in genetic value of animals, reduction in loss from parasitism and disease, and improvements in the regularity, quantity and quality of feed. Improved standards of management and housing have also contributed.

Over a slightly shorter period (1955 - 85) the same authors show that labour productivity in livestock production increased more than seven-fold, with the greatest gains in the dairy and poultry sectors.

Parallel improvements in factor productivity have taken place in European livestock production. These changes have been accompanied by steady increases in the size of economic units. Together, these two factors have enabled producers to continue production in the face of a long term decline of the order of 3% per annum in real product prices.

Position in World Trade

For all livestock products except sheep meat, the European Union is a net exporter. In the year 2000, self-sufficiency levels were 107% for pig meat, 103% for beef, 109% for poultry meat, 81% for sheep meat and 108% for dairy products. This production beyond the

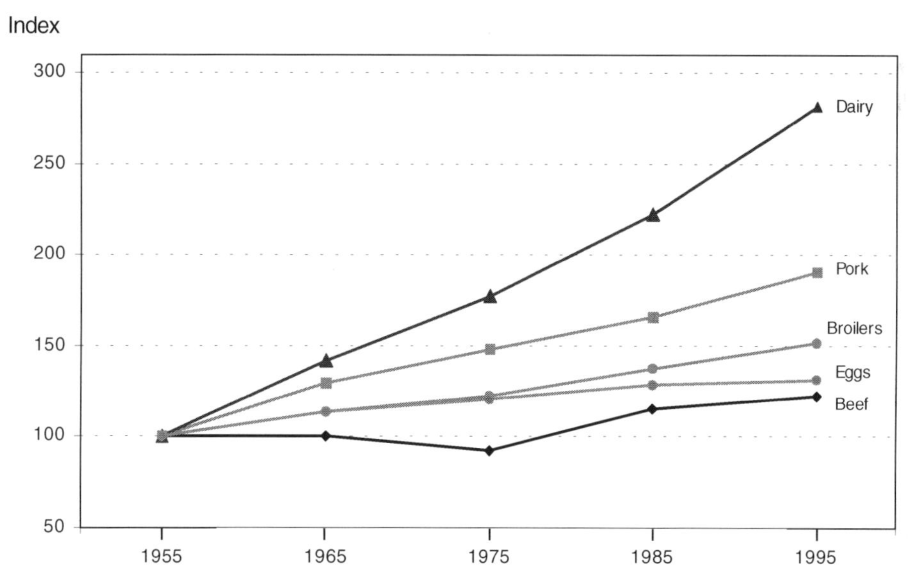

Figure 2.12. Productivity growth in US livestock production 1955 - 1995, beef: kg/cow; pork: kg/sow; milk: kg/cow, broilers: kg/bird; eggs: eggs/bird/year (Source: Fuglie et al 2000).

requirements of the internal market is a modest proportion of total output. In 2000, with a total meat production of 38.2 million tonnes, the market surplus was 2.14 million tonnes or 5.6% of production.

Most of these surpluses are exported to world markets, and most of these exports are subsidised. The future of the European livestock sector will depend heavily on how these exportable surpluses are dealt with in future years, as well as on the effect that global trading patterns and arrangements will have on competition on the internal market.

In terms of total trade in agricultural products, the EU is a net importer, with exports of temperate zone products more than balanced by imports of tropical products. The bulk of exports are to other parts of the developed world (North America 22%, Asia, including Japan 13%, CEEC 10%). A small proportion (7%) goes to the 77 ACP (African, Caribbean and Pacific) countries, which include nearly all the poorest economies in the world.

For the principal livestock products, from 4% to 11% of global production enters international trade. The figures for 1999 are shown in **Table 2.8**.

For dairy products, the EU provides about a quarter of global exports, and for meat about 20%. European exports are therefore substantial, but not dominant in the market.

Negotiations under the WTO to reduce, and eventually eliminate, distortions in global trade in agricultural products are proceeding, though with considerable uncertainty following the proposals of the 2002 US Farm Bill.

A number of studies have attempted to quantify the economic impact of such distortions, and to predict the consequences of their reduction or elimination. A recent study (Borrell & Hubbard 2000) uses a general equilibrium model of the world's most important economies to simulate what would happen if the CAP were abolished, and EU barriers to trade and direct subsidies were eliminated. Many assumptions are involved, though these are based on "reasonable empirical estimates of historical producer and consumer economic behaviour".

The study concludes that the current CAP regime sustains European grain and milk production at levels more than 50% higher than would be the case under fully liberalised

Table 2.8 EU and World trade in livestock products 1999 (Source: European Commission 2001)

		% of World Trade	
	% of world output traded	Imported by EU	Exported by EU
Butter	11	16.4	20.5
Cheese	8	13.0	31.9
Milk powder	45	3.2	32.0
Meat (total)	7	7.6	20.4
Beef	10	7.1	16.7
Pigmeat	4	2.4	41.6
Poultry meat	10	5.8	15.7

trading. For livestock and meat products, the corresponding figures were 30% and 18%. These figures therefore represent, in broad terms, one set of potential consequences of full global trade liberalisation: reduced EU prices, leading to about one third reduction in the scale of the grain and dairy sectors, and about one fifth in the meat sector.

The net effect would be to turn the EU from being an exporter of these products into being the world's largest importer. This, they calculate, would lead to an increase of up to 38% in global prices, which in turn would stimulate increased output in other economies.

Effects on developing countries

For some developing countries, the availability of low cost subsidised imports, particularly of grain and milk products, can be advantageous. In other cases, competition from subsidised imports undermines the viability of local production, and therefore hinders development. The overall balance of benefit and damage is difficult to establish, but cases where the disposal of European surplus inhibits the development opportunities for poor countries will undoubtedly not be tolerable in future years.

There is a high degree of dependence on agriculture in developing countries where the average share of agriculture in GDP is about 25% and agricultural exports account for more than one-third of export earnings.

As agricultural exports are strongly and positively correlated with economic growth (Scandizzo 1998), one of the key concerns is access to competitive markets. Agricultural policies largely determine this access, and recently it has been estimated that developing countries could carry annual welfare losses of $20bn a year as a result of industrialised countries' agricultural policies (World Bank 2001b).

Since 1992 CAP reforms in the EU have progressively decreased trade-distorting subsidies, making some headway towards reducing inequalities in world trade to the benefit of all suppliers, including developing country suppliers. Export subsidies now represent 8% of the CAP budget, and 5.2% of the value of farm exports as compared to 30% in 1991.

In its most recent proposals (December 2002) for the WTO, the EU indicated its intention to further reduce export subsidies by 45% and trade distorting domestic support by 55%. Currently, 97% of LDC exports enter the EU duty free. The new proposal will provide for 100% duty and quota free access for all farm imports from LDC countries.

While there have been specific cases where European export practices inhibit local production in poor countries, these cases are exceptions in a pattern of EU - LDC trade that is broadly and progressively complementary.

For the future of the European livestock sector, these issues of equity in trade relations with the developing world are unlikely to be a major factor. In the first place, livestock products are a very small part of this trade. In the years 1996 - 99, products of livestock origin made up just 0.84% of agricultural exports of LDCs and 8.94% of their imports (Diaz-Bonilla et al, 2002). More broadly, the proposed changes in the CAP, together with initiatives to make trading arrangements more favourable to developing countries are likely to progressively remove these issues from the political and economic agenda.

2.9 Evolution of EU Common Agricultural Policy

The foundation document of the European Community, the Treaty of Rome (1958), defined the general objectives of a Common Agricultural Policy (CAP). The principles of the CAP were set out at the Stresa Conference in July 1958. In 1960, the CAP mechanisms were adopted by the six founding member states, and two years later, in 1962, the CAP came into force. The policy created a single market for agricultural products, and provided for financial solidarity through a European Agricultural Guidance and Guarantee Fund (EAGGF).

In the forty years since then, the CAP has broadly fulfilled its declared objectives. These objectives [Article 33 (39) of the EC Treaty] are:

- to increase agricultural productivity by promoting technical progress and by ensuring the rational development of agricultural production and the optimum utilization of the factors of production, in particular labour;
- thus to ensure a fair standard of living for the agricultural community, in particular by increasing the individual earnings of persons engaged in agriculture;
- to stabilize markets;
- to assure the availability of supplies; and
- to ensure that supplies reach consumers at reasonable prices.

At the same time, as the Community was progressively enlarged, and became the European Union, and as the economic structure of European countries has developed, a number of reforms of the CAP have been implemented. The first major reform, known as the Mansholt Plan (1968) sought to reduce the number of people employed in agriculture, and to promote the formation of larger and more efficient units of production.

Despite continued structural changes in the following years, problems persisted; the supply and demand of agricultural products were not in balance, resulting in ever growing surpluses. The budgetary cost of the CAP (at that time 72% of total EC budget) was also a matter of continuing attention. In 1985, the Commission issued a Green Paper "Perspectives for the Common Agricultural Policy", and in 1988 a new reform (The Delors 1 Package), reforming the financial system and CAP and doubling structural funds, was agreed.

A further cycle of reforms (The MacSharry Package) was enacted in 1992. This provided for a reduction in agricultural prices to render them more competitive in the internal and world markets, with compensation of farmers for loss of income, as well as other measures related to market mechanisms and protection of the environment. At the same time, the inclusion of agriculture for the first time in the General Agreement on Tariffs and Trade (GATT) introduced further pressures in the same direction.

These trends culminated in the implementation of Agenda 2000, the most radical and comprehensive reform of the CAP since its inception. This reform provided for

- the reinforcement of the competitiveness of agricultural commodities in domestic and world markets;
- the promotion of a fair and decent standard of living for the farming community;
- the creation of substitute jobs and other sources of income for farmers;
- the formation of a new policy for rural development, which becomes the second pillar of the CAP;
- the integration of more environmental and structural considerations into the CAP;
- the improvement of food quality and safety; and

- the simplification of agricultural legislation and the decentralisation of its application, in order to make rules and regulations clearer, more transparent and easier to access.

The initiatives put in place under Agenda 2000 were intended to underpin EU agricultural policy until 2006. However, in July 2002, the European Commission, as part of the mid-term review of this programme, have proposed a further major cycle of reforms.

In this mid-term review, the Commission recognises that public expenditure for the farm sector must be better justified. Besides supporting farming incomes, it must yield more in return regarding food quality, the preservation of the environment and animal welfare, landscapes, cultural heritage, enhancing social balance and equity. The review is intended to reduce bureaucratic procedures, and to encourage farmers to produce at high standards for the highest market return, rather than for the sake of the maximum possible subsidy. For European consumers and taxpayers, the review will ensure better value for money. To achieve those goals, the Commission proposes:

- to cut the link between production and direct payments;
- to make those payments conditional on environmental, food safety, animal welfare and occupational safety standards;
- to substantially increase EU support for rural development via a modulation of direct payments with the exemption of small farmers;
- to introduce a new farm audit system; and
- new rural development measures to boost quality production, food safety, animal welfare and to cover the costs of the farm audit.

The broad aims of the evolving CAP are to strike a reasonable balance between the interests of the various stakeholders in the food production chain. The principal element in this balance is to serve the interests of the general public, both as consumers and taxpayers, on the one hand, and those of farmers, as food producers and custodians of the rural environment, on the other. External factors which have a bearing on this balancing exercise include commitments under the WTO, as well as the process of adaptation in the European Union to accommodate new member countries. As the number of producers (and particularly full time producers) declines, and as the demands of consumers increase, this balance, in economic terms, is progressively shifting to the disadvantage of producers. In the coming decades, it is difficult to see a reversal of this trend.

2.10 Enlargement of the EU

One of the major challenges facing the EU as a whole, and the agricultural sector in particular, is the accession of ten new states in the coming years. Along with the other adjustments required to meet changing times, the CAP, originally designed for six member states, and now serving fifteen, must be updated to accommodate the needs of twenty five states.

The ten central and Eastern European Countries (CEEC) now on track for membership have a very different agricultural structure from the current EU. **Table 2.9** summarises some key statistics.

Despite the fact that these countries experienced, in varying degrees, forty years of collectivised or state managed agriculture, the current structures in many ways resemble those of western Europe more than fifty years ago. The new CAP must therefore assist these countries in the difficult social and economic restructuring which is already two generations advanced in the rest of the EU.

Table 2.9 EU15 and the 10 CEEC accession countries - general and agricultural statistics (1997).

	EU15	CEEC10	CEEC as % of EU
Population (m)	373	105	28
GDP/head (Euro)	18 154	5 118	28
Employed in agriculture (m)	7.5	10	133
Agric. Area (m Ha)	135	60	44
Agric. as % of GDP	1.7	7	412
Agric. as % of Employment	5.1	22.5	441
Food expediture as % of household income	18	23-58	
Arable land (m Ha)	76	41	54
Cattle (m)	84	17	20
Cows (m)	34	8	24
Pigs (m)	118	41	35
Sheep (m)	94	16	17

(Source: Agricultural Situation and Prospects in the Central and Eastern European Countries, Summary Report, European Commission, June 1998).

Just how challenging this task will be is clear from the statistical comparison. Despite having a total population one quarter as large as that in EU15, the CEEC have 33% more people employed in agriculture: 10 million as against 7.5 million. Productivity levels are low, and therefore economic output per person employed in agriculture is only 11% of that in the western countries. Real incomes in society are one third of those in the EU.

In the post communist era, livestock numbers were reduced drastically, with the result that the livestock sector in CEEC is smaller than its historical levels. Despite this, and despite the fact that output per animal and per hectare are lower than in EU15, the CEEC also face problems of surplus production in all livestock products and in cereals. The adjustment process must therefore take place without the advantage of a growing internal market, as was the case during much of the comparable evolution in western Europe.

References

Anderson K., Dimaranan A., Francois J., Hertel T., Hoekman B., Martin W. (2001). *The cost of rich (and poor) country protection to developing countries.* CIES Discussion Paper No 0136. Adelaide, Centre for International Economic Studies.

Atkinson N. (2001). The Impact of BSE on the UK Economy. *MAFF UK Paper,* presented at IICA; *www.iica.org.ar/BSE/14-%20Atkinson.html*

Basnet B.B., Apan A.A., *et al.* (2002). Geographic information system based manure application plan. *Journal of Environmental Management* 64: 99-113.

Benet J.J. (1999). *La tuberculose.* Document support de cours aux étudiants des écoles nationales vétérinaires, 152 pp.

Biering-Sorensen U. (1959). *Ophobning af tilfaelde af avier tuberkulose* I en svinebesaetning. Medd Dan Dyrlaegeforen, 42, 550-552

Bindraban, P. S., J. J. Stoorvogel, *et al.* (2000). Land quality indicators for sustainable land management : proposed method for yield gap and soil nutrient balance. *Agriculture, Ecosystems and Environment* 81: 103-112.

Blancou J. (2000). Histoire de la surveillance et du contrôle des maladies animales transmissibles. *Office International des Epizooties OIE éd.* 366 pp.

Borrell B. & Hubbard L.J. (2000). Global economic effects of the EU Common Agricultural Policy, *Economic Affairs*, 20, 18-26

Boyle G.E., Brown S. & O'Regan K. (2002). *The Competitiveness of Irish Agriculture*, The Irish Farmers Journal (in press).

Danish Cattle Federation. (2002). Annual Report, *www.lr.dk*.

De Haan C., Steinfeld H. & Blackburn H. (1998). *Livestock and the environment, finding a balance*. Wren Media Fressingfield, UK.

DEFRA, Department for the Environment, Food and Rural Affairs, UK, *www.defra.gov.uk*

Diaz-Bonnilla E., Robinson S., Thomas M. & Yanoma Y. (2002). WTO, Agriculture,and Developing Countries: A survey of issues. *TMD Discussion* Paper No. 81, IFPRI, Washington

EEA, European Environment Agency. (2002). Agriculture. Chapter 7 In: *Environmental Signals 2001*. Environmental Assessment Report. No. 8: 49-56. *http://eea.eu.int*

ERS, USDA, Economic Research Service of the United States Department of Agriculture; *www.ers.usda.gov/*

European Commission. (2000). *Agenda 2000: for a stronger and wider Union, European Commission http://europa.eu.int/comm/agenda2000/*

European Commission. (2001). *Agricultural Situation in the European Union* from Agriculture in the European Union Statistical and Economic Information 2001 *http://europa.eu.int/comm/agriculture/agrista/2000/table_en/*

Eurostat, *Statistical Office of the European Commission http://europa.eu.int/comm/eurostat/*

FAO. (2002). *Agriculture towards 2015/30*. Rome, Food and Agriculture Organization.

Food Ethics Council. (2001). *Farming Animals for Food: Towards a Moral Menu*. Southwell, Notts, UK.

Frawley J. & Phelan G. (2002). *Changing agriculture: Impact on rural development*. Teagasc, Ireland *www.teagasc.ie/publications/2002/*

Fuchs F. (1968). Schweinepest. In *Handbuch der virus-infectionen bei Tieren*, Band 3 Röhrer H. ed., Jena. Gustav Fisher, P16

Fuglie K, Narrod C., & Neumeyer C. (2000). Public and private investment in Animal research In: *Public-Private Collaboration in Agricultural Research: New Institutional Arrangements and Economic Implications*.Fuglie K. & D. Schimmelpfennig (Eds). Iowa State Press.

Gerber P., Chilonda P., *et al.* (2002). *Livestock density and nutrient balances across Asia.* (In press). www.ramiran.sk..

Glynn M.K., Bopp C., Dewitt W., Dabney P., Mokhtar M., Angulo F.J. (1998). Emergence of multidrug-resistant Salmonella enterica serotype typhimurium DT104 infections in the United States. *N Engl J Med.* 7; 338(19):1333-8.

Goodwin R.F.W. & Jennings A.R. (1958). A highly infectious gastroenteritis of pigs. *Vet. Rec.* 70, 271-272

Hamscher G., SczesnyS., *et al.* (2000). *Tetracycline and chlortetracycline residues in soil fertilized with liquid manure.* Workshop 4 on sustainable animal production, Hannover.

Henderson W.M. (1978). An historical review of the control of Foot-and-Mouth disease. *Br. Vet. J.*, 134, 3-9

Hoffmann M., JohnssonH., *et al.* (2000). Leaching of nitrogen in Swedish agriculture - a historical perspective. *Agriculture, Ecosystems and Environment* 80: 227-290.

Hooda P. S., Edwards A.C., *et al.* (2000). A review of water quality concerns in livestock farming areas. *The Science of the Total Environment* 250: 143-167.

Hoppe R., Johnson J., Perry J., Korb P., Sommer J., Ryan J., Green R, Durst R., & Monke J. (2001) Structural and Financial Characteristics of US Farms: 2001 Family Farm Report. *Agriculture Information Bulletin* No.768, Resource Economics Division, Economic Research Service, US Department of Agriculture, May 2001.

International Fertiliser Industry Association (2000). *Nitrogen - Phosphate - Potash IFADATA statistics from 1972/74 - 1998/99.* Paris, France.

ITC, International Trade Centre. (2002). *Overview world markets for organic food & beverages (estimates).* UNCTAD/WTO.

Mead P.S., Slutsker L., Dietz V., McCaig L.F., Bresee J.S., Shapiro C., Griffin P.M. & Tauxe R.V. (1999). Food-related illness and death in the United States. *Emerging Infectious Diseases.* 5(5): 607-25.

Milne L.M., Bhagani S., Bannister B.A., Laitner S.M., Moore P., Eza D. & Chodini P.L. (2001). Trichinellosis acquired in the United Kingdom. *Epidemiology and Infection*, 127, 359-363

OECD. (2001). OECD national soil surface nitrogen balances, *OECD*: 19.

OECD, Organisation for Economic Co-operation and Development, Main Economic Indicators. *www.oecd.org/statistics/*

Oxfam. (2002). Market access and agricultural trade: the double standards of rich countries Chapter 4 In: *Rigged rules and double standards: trade, globalisation and the fight against poverty.* Oxford, Oxfam. *www.maketradefair.com*

Plowright W. (1965). Rinderpest, *Vet. Rec.* 77, 1431-1438

Pretty J.N., Brett C., Gee D., Hine R.E., Mason C.F., Morison J.I.L., Raven H., Rayment M.D., & van der Bijl G., (2000). An assessment of the total external costs of UK agriculture. *Agricultural Systems* 65: 113-136.

Scandizzo P.L. (1998). *Growth, trade and agriculture: An investigative survey.* FAO Economic and Social Development Paper 143. Rome, Food and Agriculture Organization.

Schröder J. (2002). *Restoring farmer's confidence in manure benefits the environment.* (In press), www.ramiran.sk

Scoones I. & Toulmin C. (1998). Soil nutrient balances: what use for policy? *Agriculture, Ecosystems and Environment* 71: 255-267.

Truyen U., Parrish C.R., Harder T.C. & Kaaden O.R. (1995). There is nothing permanent except change: the emergence of new diseases. *Vet. Microbiol.* 43, 103-122

USDA. (2002a). Captive supply of cattle and GIPSA's reporting of captive supply. 63 pp. *USDA Report,* January 2002

USDA. (2002b). United State Department of Agriculture, Farm Bill 2002 *www.usda.gov/farmbill/*

Uunk E.J.B. (1991). *Eutrophication of surface waters and the contribution of agriculture.* London, The Fertiliser Society.

World Bank. (2001a). Global Economic Prospects and the Developing countries 2001. Washington, World Bank

World Bank. (2001b). World Development Report: Attacking Poverty. Washington, World Bank.

Chapter 3. The Future: Vision and Options

The BSE crisis has signalled the need for a fundamental reappraisal of the animal production industry's priorities and practices. Formulating a vision for a new European industry will require inputs from all interested parties – citizens, politicians, farmers, retailers, scientists and economists, as well as from those actively engaged in the agri-food industry. It is unlikely that the invisible hand of the market will suffice, for "where there is no vision, the people perish" (Proverbs 26; 18). In every country in Europe, as well as at EU level, this search for a new vision of agriculture and food production is being pursued.

In many cases, the debate leads to a conclusion that much of recent and current development should be reversed. This conclusion is well articulated in a recent report on UK farming and food (Curry, 2002). The authors say "our central theme is reconnection ... the key objective of public policy should be to reconnect our food and farming industry: to reconnect farming with its market and the rest of the food chain; to reconnect the food chain and the countryside; and to reconnect consumers with what they eat and how it is produced". Similar conclusions can be found in other reports at national level, for example, in The Netherlands (Netherlands Ministry of Agriculture, 2001).

The vision includes:

- Decoupling support payments from products and shifting support to sustainable rural development;
- Returning to more ecologically balanced mixed farming systems; and
- Shortening and promoting reconnection in the food chain.

Carrying such a vision forward presents great challenges. Perhaps the greatest is that the industry is in many ways driven in the opposite direction by economic forces. The relentless downward pressure on output prices can only be met by steady increases in the scale, efficiency, and often the intensification, of production.

Furthermore, the great national and international corporations that now control most of food processing and distribution are not comfortable partners for large numbers of widely dispersed family-owned farm enterprises. Power in the food chain has shifted to the corporations. While farmers and food corporations do have interests in common - most clearly in ensuring that the ultimate consumer has confidence in food quality and safety - they also have interests that are in very direct conflict. These largely concern the trading relationships between the two sides. The corporations buy their raw material from the farmers. Corporate selling prices to consumers are under continuous competitive pressure. In addition, increasingly complex manufacturing and distribution systems, and growing regulatory requirements, add to their costs. Corporate profits are best maintained by passing these pressures down the line to producers. Farmers are at the end of the line. Hence the recurring state of economic crisis at farm level.

In this section elements of the vision of a "leaner, greener European model of agriculture, with contented consumers, cleaner countryside and competitive farmers" are developed.

In parallel, the ways in which this can be achieved while increasing technical and economic efficiency in the industry are explored.

The section begins with two analyses of the stakeholders and their concerns. The first takes a broad view of society's expectations from the industry. The second follows the structure of the market and reflects the economic relationship between the various sectors.

3.1 Stakeholders - The Ethical Framework

A number of measures necessary in the short to medium-term have been recommended to manage the BSE epidemic in Europe and to restore public confidence in the safety of food and other products derived from cattle. While such measures are necessary they are by no means sufficient. BSE was symptomatic of a much larger problem, which has become evident for instance in the more recent outbreaks of CSF and FMD.

There is evidence that public concerns over animal products are much wider and more fundamental than those impacting on human safety and food prices. They extend to animal welfare, protection of the environment, rebuilding consumer trust and the need to ensure fairness in respect of the consequences of international trade. In short, importance is increasingly being assigned to the ethics of animal production systems.

The examination of the many issues and interests affected by BSE has been informed by implicit appeal to a set of ethical principles. Those principles have been used to construct a framework called the "ethical matrix" (Mepham 2000) and used in studies of the UK livestock sector (Food Ethics Council 2001a, 2001b).

Despite the increasing diversity of modern multicultural, pluralistic societies, the pursuit of democracy would seem to make certain assumptions that conform to the idea of a 'common morality'. These assumptions are encapsulated by three *prima facie* principles, namely, respect for:

- well-being
- autonomy
- justice

Appeal to these principles does not determine the outcome of ethical reasoning, but it does ensure that attention is paid to a range of relevant issues, that a consistent approach is adopted and that any decisions made are explicit. The principles are based on established ethical theories (utilitarianism, Kantianism and the Rawlsian theory of 'justice as fairness') that commonly feature in perceptions of 'rightful actions'. The importance attached to such principles may differ between people, but for most people concern for well-being, autonomy and justice *matters* – not only for themselves but also for others, whether human or non-human.

When they were introduced in the context of medical practice (Beauchamp & Childress 1994), they referred primarily to the interests of patients and healthcare workers, but in considering agricultural practices the issues raised have been explored by applying them to the interests of four, broadly defined, 'groups'. These are:

- People who work in the agricultural and food industries (e.g. farmers, agricultural suppliers, food manufacturers, retailers, traders and caterers);
- Citizens (all of us, both as consumers and as participants in democratic society);
- Farm animals; and

Table 3.1. An Ethical Matrix.

	WELLBEING	AUTONOMY	JUSTICE
PEOPLE IN THE AGRICULTURAL AND FOOD INDUSTRIES	Satisfactory income and working conditions	Appropriate freedom of action	Fair trade laws And practices
CITIZENS	Food safety and acceptability & Quality of life	Democratic, informed choice e.g. of food	Availability of affordable food
FARM ANIMALS	Animal welfare	Behavioural freedom	Intrinsic value
THE ECOSYSTEM	Conservation	Biodiversity	Sustainability

An ethical matrix showing, in twelve individual cells, the interpretation of respect for the principles of well-being, autonomy and justice in terms appropriate to the interests of people working in the agricultural and food industries, citizens, farm animals and the ecosystem. For people, both impacts and responsibilities are involved, whereas for farm animals and the ecosystem (shaded) only impacts of human actions are relevant.

- The Ecosystem: encompassing all organisms (including the human population, domesticated and wild species) considered collectively, as interrelated species, breeds and populations.

Because the three principles can be applied to all four interest groups, the resulting twelve types of ethical impact can be represented in the form of a table (an ethical matrix), which aims to facilitate discussion of the issues by arranging them in a rational structure (**Table 3.1**). The translations (or 'specifications') of the abstract principles are expressed in terms that are intended to be familiar but at the same time authentic from an ethical perspective. For example, respect for farm animal well-being is translated as *animal welfare*, that for citizens' autonomy is interpreted in terms of *democratic, informed choice*, and that for justice for the ecosystem as *sustainability*.

These sometimes rather imaginative interpretations are of course open to challenge and debate. However, the value of the approach has been confirmed in several exercises in public participation, at which the merits and usefulness of the matrix have been commended.

It would be a mistake to imagine that one can resolve complex ethical issues simply by consigning them to the separate 'cells' of the matrix. At its simplest, it merely serves as a check-list of concerns, which happen to be based on ethical theory. But it can also structure ways of systematically addressing the issues and serve as a means of promoting public awareness and stimulating ethical deliberation. The necessity to consider how narrow sectarian interests interact with the whole enterprise can only have beneficial effects.

3.2 Stakeholders - the Market Structure

The stakeholder categories identified in this analysis are fairly broad and fall into two different groups. The first group follows a farm-to-table analysis, looking at how various actors along that continuum may impact the health of animals, humans and the environment. The second group looks at the various institutions involved and at the impact that they may have.

Regarding the principal concerns of the various groups of stakeholders, it is clear that in almost all cases a critical concern is economic profit. In a competitive world, such profit can be equated with economic survival. This is a real issue for livestock producers, since the farm enterprise is usually more than just a livelihood. The group with a different primary concern is consumers, for whom food price, quality and safety are paramount.

Farm-to-table stakeholders

For the purpose of this analysis the potential stakeholders are categorised into six subgroups affecting: (i) inputs into production, (ii) production (raising) of livestock, (iii) processing and preparation of livestock products, (iv) wholesalers and retailers of livestock products, (v) food service providers, and (vi) consumers. A brief description of the categories is given below.

Table 3.2 presents a list of identified stakeholders and an assessment of their potential impact on animal, human, and environmental health. Their ability to have such an impact is ranked by asterisks. Three asterisks denote major impact while one denotes only a little.

Input Providers

The principal concern of all input providers is economic profits. Suppliers of breeding material have the ability to affect animal health by developing breeding stock which has been selected for certain disease resistance traits. They can also affect animal health by using techniques for the delivery of semen or embryos which reduce the risk of disease transmission. Providers of feed and nutritional inputs can affect animal health by ensuring the delivery of disease-free feed. They also have the ability to affect human health by ensuring that feed and feed additives used do not compromise the safety of meat/milk/eggs for human consumption. Those involved in the delivery of veterinary supplies can affect animal health by ensuring the delivery of uniform, effective, and high quality vaccines and drugs. They can affect human health by ensuring that preventive medicines used in raising animals are not at levels where residuals would interfere with treatment of human diseases, or contribute to the development of resistant pathogens.

Production

As for other actors in the food chain, economic profit is a principal concern for producers. However, most producers are family farmers, whose production resources often consist of a patrimony of many generations, and include the family home.

Non-cash concerns about ensuring the survival, maintenance and integrity of the farm are therefore also a major factor.

Producers can take measures to prevent productivity losses associated with disease in their animals. They can affect human health by establishing measures that prevent microbial diseases on-farm. They can also impact environmental health by disposing of manure (or treating it) in a manner that nutrients do not overload the environment and that pathogens do not get into the human food chain (i.e. drinking water, aquaculture, fruit and vegetables).

Veterinarians safeguard animal health by identifying and treating sick/diseased animals prior to the spread of disease in a herd. They can also affect human health by identifying and treating such animals before they enter the human food chain. They can affect environmental health by preventing animal disease from farmed animal populations from getting into wild populations. Those involved in the transportation of live animals to

Table 3.2 Farm to table stakeholders.

Stakeholders	Principal health issues		
	Animal	Human	Environment
Input Providers			
Breeding Suppliers	***		
Feed/Nutritional Sector	***	**	
Veterinary Suppliers	***	**	
Production			
On farm	***	**	**
Veterinary services	***	**	*
Animal transport	***	*	
Processors			
Slaughterhouse	*	***	**
Fabrication		***	*
Packaging and transport of carcasses/prepared food		***	
Disposal of by-products of animal origin	*	**	***
Food wholesalers/retailers			
Storage/distribution/sale of carcasses/ prepared food		***	
Storage/ processing of by-products of animal origin			***
Food service providers			
Institutional food providers		***	
Restaurants		***	*
Consumers			
Different groups	*	***	*

slaughter can also affect animal and human health by identifying sick and/or diseased animals.

Processors

The main concern of most of those involved in the slaughtering and fabrication of animals is also economic profits. They can affect human health by preventing product from diseased animals from getting into the human food chain. They can also control and reduce microbial contamination at all stages. They can affect environmental health by treating by-products prior to disposal and by recycling by-products whenever possible. Transport may be the responsibility of the slaughterhouse or the wholesaler/retailer or it may be by private operators. During this stage, growth of microbial pathogens can take place. Growth and cross-contamination of microbial pathogens can be reduced via refrigeration and measures to prevent cross contamination of carcasses during transport. Improved logistics of getting products from slaughterhouses to food wholesalers/retailers can reduce spoilage and cross contamination from contaminated carcasses. Those involved in the disposal of by-products of animal origin can affect animal health by making sure that any potentially contaminated risk material is prevented from getting into the animal feed chain. They can also affect animal, human, and environmental health by making sure that by-products are treated for pathogens and that as much nutrient content as possible is recycled prior to entry into the environment.

Food wholesalers/retailers

This group of stakeholders is dominated by the large retail supermarket firms. They are interested primarily in economic profits. Those involved in the storage and distribution of both carcasses and prepared food can make sure that the processes they use retard the growth of microbes and spoilage of food prior to human consumption. Those involved in the storage of by-products of animal origin can affect environmental health by recycling as much nutrients a possible prior to storage.

Food service providers

Similarly those involved in the delivery of foods to consumers via restaurants or institutional catering are interested primarily in making a living. Like retailers and wholesalers they can affect human health by ensuring that the processes they use retard the growth of microbes and spoilage of food prior to human consumption.

Consumers

Consumers are interested mainly in access to safe, affordable food. The trade-off between price, quality and safety depends on income levels, cultural factors and changing consumption patterns. Consumers are affected by transient events, such as food scares or periods of economic stress or prosperity. There are also many subgroups of consumers with special interests. It is therefore difficult to state a principal concern that applies across the population. It is clear, however, that consumer choice is primarily price driven. Because, for most foods at most times, there is little need to be concerned about safety, safety becomes an issue (but an over-riding one) only when consumers are alerted to potential dangers. Finally, quality of food means different things to different age, cultural and economic groups. It therefore has a very variable ranking among the three principal concerns of consumers.

Consumer impact on animal, human and environmental health will also vary across the different groups of consumers. Animal and environmental health are marginally affected, but consumer choice can have major impact on human health, for example by excessive caloric intake, excessive fat, or insufficient fibre in the diet.

Institutional stakeholders

For the purpose of this analysis institutional stakeholders are divided into two groups, those that are part of the national, provincial, and local government and those that are part of the international standard setting bodies. **Table 3.3** presents a list of identified stakeholders, their principal concerns, and an assessment of their potential impact on animal, human, and environmental health. As in Table 3.1, their ability to alter animal, human, and environmental health is ranked by asterisks.

National, provincial, and local governments

The principal concern of those in the national, provincial, and local governments is the provision of improved services that result in the protection of animal, human, and environmental health. Livestock extension services can pursue these goals by providing animal production standards, aiding farmers in adopting and meeting standards, improving labour conditions, and aiding farmers in mitigating environmental problems. Those involved in providing animal health services can safeguard animal health by enforcing animal health standards, aiding farmers in adopting and meeting standards, monitoring

Table 3.3 Institutional Stakeholders.

Stakeholders	Principal concerns	Health issues		
		Animal	Human	Environment
National, provincial, and local governments				
Livestock Extension	Improved animal production	***	*	**
Animal Health/ Welfare Services	Improved animal health and welfare	***		
Meat Inspection Service	Identify disease of human health concern	*	***	
Food Safety Agency	Safeguard human health		***	
Environmental Protection Agency	Improved Environment			***
International standard setting bodies				
OIE	Reduce livestock disease worldwide	***		
CODEX	Reduce food borne disease worldwide		***	

and enforcing compliance, and preventing the spread of disease. Similarly (and this can also be a responsibility of the animal health service) there is a role in monitoring and enforcing compliance of animal welfare standards.

In the wake of the BSE and other crises of confidence in the food industry, many governments (and the EU) have set up new food safety institutions. Such food safety agencies can affect human health by providing standards and aiding participants along the farm to table chain in adopting and meeting these standards. They can also improve human health by monitoring and enforcing compliance to standards, as well as by educating consumers, food service workers and industry managers in guaranteed delivery of safe food to consumers. Environmental protection agencies can improve environmental health by providing standards, aiding farmers and processors in adopting and meeting these standards, and monitoring and enforcing compliance to environmental regulations.

International standard setting bodies concerned with animal and human health

The principal concern of the international standard setting bodies is to aid countries in their efforts to reduce livestock disease and food-borne human disease world-wide. OIE is the WTO standard setting body with regard to animal health. Their goal is to limit the spread of disease via trade and to monitor disease outbreaks worldwide. Recently OIE has decided to broaden its spectrum to animal welfare and to certain aspects of food safety. CODEX is the standard setting body with regard to food safety worldwide.

3.3 The Economic Context

As in other sectors of the economy, change in the livestock sector is ultimately driven by economic forces. Policies developed through a political process are put into action through financial incentives or disincentives. Within such a policy framework, market forces determine the structure of the industry.

In all countries, and strongly in the European Union, the policy framework has had very explicit social as well as economic objectives. The result has been a sequence of policies designed both to promote change toward increased economic efficiency and to moderate change in the interest of maintaining the viability of rural livelihoods. To a considerable degree, these aims are contradictory. The result is that neither aim is ever fully realised.

Whatever changes in policy there are, whether driven by internal political initiative or by external pressures through the WTO, this dilemma will persist. At its centre is the reality that the unit scale of a majority of European livestock producers is too small for economic viability. Three quarters of the 7 million farms in the EU do not provide for one full employment position. With the imminent enlargement, there will be an additional 10 million farmers, the great majority of them below this threshold.

This central issue of scale is not directly resolvable in either economic or social terms. In particular, any attempt to measure scale in European livestock production on the same basis as in some other developed economies is unrealistic. US producers have eight times the land resources on average, Australian producers 65 times (Table 2.4). Yet, in both of these economies, producers are in recurrent crisis, and family scale production is only marginally viable.

What then should Europe do on the scale issue? At national and at EU level many policies and programmes are already in place to sustain rural livelihoods, to stimulate off-farm employment, and to promote steady increases in efficiency and quality of production. Much emphasis is given now to the social value of countryside maintenance. The move towards decoupling of support from production is now widely accepted. In the livestock sector, some specific additional initiatives are possible.

Where production has a quota structure (primarily milk) the quota entitlement has acquired a capital value (**Box 7**). For small, sub-economic, quota holders, it might be worthwhile to buy in and extinguish the quota entitlement. This could provide a capital incentive for transition to other work, either on farm or off. It would also reduce market surpluses, and consolidate the industry into more viable units.

The age profile of the livestock producers in all European countries shows a preponderance of older farmers. Most are content to continue in farming. In order to discourage their potential successors from continuing with production on an uneconomic scale, a specific programme of education for alternative career paths might be productive. In many cases this might effectively be training for off-farm employment, while supporting the rural structure and current land tenure system through a move to part time, and perhaps less intensive, production.

Box 7. Dairy Quotas

Dairy production is in several respects the most important element in the EU livestock sector. With 642,000 producers, most of whom are full time, it is the largest provider of on-farm employment. Milk sales represent 14% of gross agricultural output, and dairy farms are the source of more than half of the beef output, which adds a further 10%.

To regulate persistent and growing surpluses, a quota system was introduced in 1984. Initially opposed by most dairy farmers, quotas are now defended for the stability and protection that they give to producers.

Within the common EU rules, the management of the quota system varies somewhat between countries. The impact of the system can be illustrated by the case of Ireland. The country's 28,000 dairy farmers have an average quota of about 180,000 litres. This corresponds to an average dairy herd size of 40 cows. Production is grass based, with low (800 kg) concentrate inputs. For the average holder, milk represents 72% of gross farm output, and production costs exceed 60% of output value. At the current price of 28 cents per litre, this gives a farmer with an average quota an income of €28,000. This slightly exceeds the average industrial wage for the country (€26,945). About 60% of producers have quotas below the average, and therefore dairy incomes below the average industrial wage. This comparison does not take account of the owned land and other capital involved in the dairy enterprise.

Since their inception, quotas have become progressively more tradable, and have acquired a capital value, currently 34 cents per litre. The possibility of selling quota is an additional incentive for those who wish to cease production. At present, about 6% do so each year. Most of these are smaller producers. The system can therefore claim both to offer stability to producers and to promote consolidation of the industry into more viable units for the future.

Livestock production is increasingly embedded in a complex of interconnected economic sectors. Its raw materials and products are traded internationally. As with other sectors of the global economy, it must compete both for access to its inputs and for markets for its outputs. In future years, tightening access to energy sources may impact the sector. Recent studies (**Box 8**) have documented the extent of reliance on fossil energy in modern cereal and livestock production, as well as the likelihood of substantial pressure on oil supplies.

3.4 Reconnecting the Chain

The Foot and Mouth Disease (FMD) epidemic of 2000 provoked widespread public concern with farming systems in the UK, particularly with the production end of the food chain. This deep concern has fed upon anxiety about the BSE epidemic.

Following the FMD epidemic several commissions were established to make recommendations on different aspects of the outbreak. The report of the first Policy Commission on the Future of Farming and Agriculture (Curry, 2002) concluded unequivocally that the present system of farming is unsustainable. Radical change is absolutely necessary. Turning around a great industry however takes time, courage, vision and co-operation. Simply going in the opposite direction is not a solution.

The Curry Report strongly advocates connectedness as a theme to resolve the current lack of consumer confidence. In effect, The report notes that the food chain is not a chain but rather a series of components which are not adequately linked, are focused on their own specific interests, and that decision-making in each component is highly motivated by efficiency within that sector. The report recommends reconnection: reconnecting farmers with their market and the rest of the food chain; the food chain with a healthy and attractive countryside; and consumers with what they eat and where it has come from.

Translating such a theme into practice is not easy. Although the food chain is efficient in economic terms, measured by the unit cost of food, in the short-term use of natural resources and in the interests of the owners of the components in the middle of the chain - the processors, transporters, industries supplying supporting resources such as packaging and advertising and of course the outlets, especially supermarkets characterized by competition for consumer attention and among each other – producers at the end of the chain are marginalized. The principal way for producers to survive is to increase the scale of production units, in turn often leading to increasing intensification. Small farmers cannot compete. This has a major impact upon rural development, unemployment in rural areas and quality of life in the countryside.

The lack of connectedness diagnosed by the Curry Report reflects the need for recognition of community in the food chain. This does not imply replacing sound business practice with some other social system. It means recognising that each link in the food chain and the whole of society gain or lose together. Events like FMD and BSE negatively affect all sectors in the food chain. The costs of such disasters can quickly offset years of economic benefits gained by actions such as the feeding of meat and bone meal.

Establishing connectedness requires co-operation in the better identification of food resources and products. Despite the efficiency of the food chain in reducing the unit costs of food, the source and nature of food products must also be known. A system where the primary product - milk, beef, pork - disappears into a trading network, loses its

Box 8. Energy Use and Livestock Production

Though primary agriculture uses only 5% of global consumption of fossil energy (Pinstrup-Andersen, 1999), modern grain production, and therefore industrialised systems of livestock production, are highly dependent on fossil fuels. The future of Europe's livestock sector is therefore linked to the availability and cost of oil.

While the real price of oil has declined substantially from the peaks of the 70s and 80s, in the longer term it is likely to rise. Analysis of known and probable reserves and extraction rates indicate that global production will begin an irreversible decline about a decade from now (Hatfield, 1997; Campbell, 2000). While natural gas and coal reserves will last much longer, their use as substitutes for oil will involve cost increases. It is likely therefore that intensive livestock production systems dependent on grain will also face major cost increases.

Analyses of energy use in modern cereal production have produced figures ranging from 2.7 (Dalgaard *et al.*, 2001) to 5.02 (Pimentel, 2001) and 5.27 (Sainz, 2002) MJ of fossil energy input per kg of grain output. These figures are equivalent to 77, 144 and 151 litres of diesel equivalent per ton of grain.

In most modern livestock systems, energy is also needed for transport, heating or cooling buildings, and for processing the products. These additional energy inputs may exceed those required for feed production. For example, it has been calculated (Sainz, 2002) that the energy required in modern broiler systems is approximately 32 MJ per kg of carcass weight produced, equivalent to 0.89 litres of diesel. Some 46% of this energy is for the feed component. Refsgaard et al. (1998) found total direct and indirect energy use on Danish dairy farms to be between 2.2 and 3.6 MJ per kg of milk depending on farming system and soil type. These figures were confirmed by Halberg (1999) who demonstrated that the variation between farms is a possibility for improvements by changed farm management. Energy costs in pig production on four farms was between 14 and 20 MJ per kg liveweight gain, also with systematic differences between farms over three years.

References

Campbell C.J. (2000). The imminent oil crisis. Proceedings of the Clean Energy 2000 Conference, Geneva.

Dalgaard T. *et al.* (2001). A model for fossil energy use in Danish agriculture used to compare basic organic and conventional farming. LPS, No 87 pp. 51-56.

Halberg N. (1999). Indicators of resource use and environmental impact for use in a decision aid for Danish livestock farmers. Agriculture, Ecosystems & Environment 76, pp. 17-30

Hatfield C.B. (1997). Oil back on the Global Agenda. Nature 387, 121.

Pimentel D. (2000). Biomass utilization, limits of. In Encyclopaedia of Physical Science and Technology. Third Edition Vol 2, p. 159.

Pinstrup-Andersen P. (1999). Towards Ecologically Sustainable World Food Production, Vol. 22. United Nations Environment Programme, Paris, pp.10-13.

Refsgaard K., Halberg N. & Kristensen E.S. (1998). Energy utilization in crop production on organic and conventional livestock farms. Agric. Systems 57, pp. 599-630.

Sainz R.D. (2002). Fossil Fuel Component. Framework for Calculating Fossil Fuel Use in Livestock Systems. Livestock Environment and Development Initiative (LEAD) Toolbox. FAO.

identity and eventually reaches the consumer with all identity lost or removed should be unacceptable.

Business organizations need to recognize that they are part of a civil society whose values include successful economics but are not limited to those values. Mechanisms need to be found by which decision-makers incorporate community values into the decision-making practices and processes of the chain.

Some efforts are now being made to facilitate better communication along the food chain. For example, the BSE and FMD outbreaks have forced governments and the EU to stress the need for traceability of animals and animal food products. This has been spear-headed by veterinary health services who are concerned about animal and animal product movements.

However, the increased security brings with it an increase in costs. Unless there is a sense of community among the participants of the food chain, these costs are likely to be passed back to the primary producers, making it more difficult for them to meet the dual aims of low costs and totally accountable production.

3.5 Transparency and Accountability

In western society, where so few people are now involved in the supply of food, there is widespread ignorance of the detailed working of the food chain. Over the last fifty years food supply has become so abundant, varied, available and cheap that it is often taken for granted.

The predictability of the demand for food has had an unusual effect on the supply organizations within the food chain. Extensive advertising, rather than persuading people to increase consumption, seeks to redirect the buyer to specific brands with claims of better quality, convenience and price.

Because consumers are certain to buy food the market is guaranteed. This is central to understanding the modern day food chain, which differs from other goods and services. As a result, the few organizations controlling the food chain are extremely powerful and relatively secure. Supermarket chains for example can negotiate low prices for bulk deliveries. Food processors negotiate with farmers the supply of raw products often years in advance with precise specification on quantity, quality and date for delivery. Farmers increasingly produce according to contracts that provide them with a degree of market security. Such contracts have built-in prices and offer an alternative to government guaranteed prices for farmers. Surviving farms become larger and more efficient while smaller scale farmers are required to find alternative goods and services for the market.

This food chain scenario has evolved under the selection pressure of reducing the unit price of food to consumers, providing convenience and processed foods in great variety and enabling business organizations at all stages of the chain to maximize profit to their shareholders. Until recently, it had been a success.

The recent BSE and FMD epidemics have changed the attitudes of consumers to the food chain. Confidence has been shaken. Consumers now realise that businesses operating the food chain have quite different values and decision-making processes to former traditional farmer-food-producers.

The absence of accountability within the food chain has created public fear and raised ethical questions about the handling of food. Governments in the EU have been criticized for a lack of concern and accountability in failing to ban the import (from the UK) and use of potentially contaminated meat and bone meal as soon as it was identified as the vector for BSE. BSE should not have been treated, as it initially was, as a national disease. The food chain is international and does not respect national borders. Malfunctions in the food chain are matters of international and public concern. Transparency and accountability in the food chain must transcend national interests, short-term profit and political expediency.

If the food chain is to become permanently more accountable and transparent, governments must be involved. In the EU, standards for traceability of food from point of origin to consumption are being introduced. Legal liability is being extended back to the primary producer

The largest integrated food market in the world, the US, manages its affairs with a reliance on federal regulation (FDA, FSIS) and on the reassuring messages of the major food companies. The negative aspects of this structure, in terms of the poor conditions of many engaged and employed in food production, the power of the corporations which control the industry, and the compromised welfare of the consumer, are well documented (Schlosser, 2001). Nevertheless, the system represents a model towards which much of the European food chain is evolving. The question is whether this evolution can be, or should be, interfered with.

The growth of corporate power seems inevitable. The recent (2002) establishment of the European Food Safety Authority (www.efsa.eu.int) is a first step in building public confidence in public surveillance of the food chain. Together with its national counterparts, the EFSA should be able to guarantee basic food safety. Thus, the two principal elements of the American model, corporate power and a strong regulatory structure, are in place in Europe.

However, Europe does not have the continental uniformity of food traditions that apply in the US. Mediterranean diets and traditions are greatly different from Nordic or Slavic. Each has deep roots in the ecology and culture of its region. These differences are part of the richness and variety that makes Europe what it is. This variety has values worth protecting. Part of the challenge for the future therefore is to find a way of acknowledging the value of Europe's diversity in the culture of food, and of ensuring that this value is reflected in political decisions.

Compulsory controls on competition in the food chain are also necessary. In 1999 the Director General of Fair Trading, UK, established a commission to examine the level and effects of competition in UK food supermarkets. The commission found significant distortions in fair competition between supermarkets and farm suppliers. For example, supermarkets were found to require farmers to contribute beyond their contract to research, advertising, packaging, hospitality and special shelf space, all of which are retailers' costs. Some supermarkets were found to require farmers to contribute lump sums for profit lost by store spoilage and by the supermarkets' own errors in forecasting demand. In these situations individual farmers are extremely vulnerable and have considerably less power than that previously provided by the co-operative system.

The UK Secretary of Trade and Industry recognised that such distortions are not acceptable. In the interests of all stakeholders, greater transparency and accountability are needed. A mandatory procedure between supermarkets and farm-suppliers has been recommended requiring the introduction of a Code of Practice, breaches of which will be dealt with by legal means. Such a code of practice was introduced in 2002 (www.oft.gov.uk).

The food chain is increasingly international in scope. The rationale for introducing civil society standards of transparency and accountability into the European food chain must also extend to trading partners. To ensure transparency and accountability beyond the EU, a comparable mechanism enforceable by law will have to be mirrored in the provisions of the WTO.

Market economy practice alone has been found incapable of anticipating and dealing with the unforeseen risk to human health posed by BSE. Damage limitation of BSE and vCJD are now the business of governments acting nationally or jointly and cannot be solved by market economy principles or organizations. It is therefore rational to conclude that, with so much at risk in the human food chain, national and international regulations requiring transparency and accountability are essential together with independent monitoring of new technologies, products and processes.

These are the minimum reasonable expectations of consumers when the control of food supply has been taken away from local communities and given to unknown distant parties whose primary values are profit. Legislated and enforceable standards of transparency and accountability in the food chain are minimum and reasonable for society to enjoy greater benefits without further tragedy from an increasingly global food chain.

3.6 Traceability

Globalisation of trade has increased the need for countries to ensure that food exports are safe and free of disease. Perceptions about quality and safety have become more important in consumer purchase decisions. The BSE outbreak sent a strong signal that more information based controls are needed, not only to protect consumers, but also to minimize possible impacts on international beef industries. Total quality assurance must ensure the safety of a product and its compliance with desired production methods and treatment of animals. Traceability has become a central theme in the resolution of food quality and safety.

There is a rapidly growing consensus in the meat industry that a fully verifiable animal identification system, that allows complete traceability from producer to consumer, is the optimal solution. Consumer confidence in bovine products will increasingly depend on full traceability (even across national borders) of animals, carcasses, meat and meat products. Through this system liability is spread to all parties in the production chain.

EU Regulation 1760/2000 requires a system for the identification and registration of bovine animals and the labelling of beef and beef products. Each animal must be labelled on both ears with identical ear tags, bearing a unique identification code, and be issued a passport containing identification code, date of birth, sex, breed or coat colour. These identifiers can be subsequently linked to central databases containing analogous information. Conventional ear tags however cannot be protected from forgery and can be exchanged by manipulation. If desired, this identification system therefore can be circumvented.

The regulation requires all fresh and frozen veal and beef to be labelled with a reference code, linking the meat to the animal of origin, the country of slaughter and cutting and the abattoir and cutting plant. Since 2002 the country of birth and countries of rearing are also required on the labels. A shortcoming of this system is that labels and/or barcodes can be separated, tampered with and removed from animals, carcasses and meat products. Errors or frauds of this nature are difficult to detect.

Governments, health agencies and disease control organizations have teamed with livestock industries, suppliers, universities, research organizations, veterinarians and technology companies to develop and implement a range of identification devices and systems. For example, electronic and radio frequency identification use electric pulses and radio waves to transmit identifiers from devices imbedded in the animals. These devices however are not fail-safe or fraud-proof. Further, they identify only whole animals and cannot be used to trace individual meat products.

Biological identification systems such as antibody assays may be more reliable. Using antibody assays, all animals in a herd, region or country are immunized with specific antigens. Later, antibody profiles can be generated from blood, urine, semen, saliva, tissue, carcass and meat and matched to a central database. Calves however do not develop antibodies until several months after birth and a proportion of animals immunized do not produce sufficient amounts of antibodies. Although not as common as in other systems, errors and fraud can occur.

A simple analytical method, which enables the independent confirmation and control of information from producers, processors and marketers is necessary. DNA analysis provides such a system (Sancristobal-Gaudy *et al.*, 2000; Cunningham & Meghen 2001). Not only can each individual be identified by its unique DNA composition but also DNA can be isolated from any source at any point in the production chain. Such innovative molecular genetic tests are already being used in forensic science and parentage testing of breeding animals.

Using modern detection methods the source animal from which a meat sample or products derived can be readily determined where initial samples have been collected from living animals. DNA profiles are matched using computer databases containing initial genotypes with almost 100% accuracy.

The main challenge is to establish an economic system to carry out separate, targeted collection, preservation, cataloguing and analysis of whole populations. Devices and methods allowing simple cost-effective collection of DNA samples are essential to this system. This can be achieved by the use of ear tagging techniques adapted to extract tissue samples.

A DNA based identification system has the following advantages:
- Forgery-free proof of origin and identity for all cattle and related products, at all stages of production;
- Stabilisation of targeted sales programmes such as organic livestock, livestock kept on national parks or livestock with special grade identification;
- Verification and monitoring of transport routes for all cattle;
- Efficient border control and international tracking of cattle;
- Reliable monitoring of epidemic control;
- Determination of quantity of beef in all (processed) foodstuffs;
- Identification of producers; and
- Identification of the animal and stock origin of milk and milk products.

It has been proposed that a tissue sample is taken from every new-born farm animal in the EU, the DNA isolated and the individual genotype stored in a central database for future reference. Consumers, retailers, dealers, butchers, processors, owners or inspectors would be in a position to verify the identity and origin of any animal or product.

The monitoring of particular groups of animals or herds for risk prevention, epidemic control or testing for illegal residues, could be immediately undertaken using such a database. If individual genotyping were consistently carried out it will be possible to react immediately to unforeseen problems providing the consumer with unparalleled protection and possibilities for monitoring. Establishing such a system in the EU would result in an enormous increase in consumer confidence in bovine products.

3.7 Consumer Assurance

With the growing number of food scares, quality assurance has become an essential aspect of: 1) the raw materials for food production, 2) the procedures involved in the productive process, and 3) the finished products.

Although food safety is a fundamental and necessary part of food quality, consumers also demand other qualitative characteristics. The consumer is becoming increasingly careful in choosing foods which are not only safe (with no health risks), but also easily digestible, tasty, energy poor, are good sources of vitamins, have essential fatty acids and trace minerals etc. and also form part of their traditional food.

Consumers would also like to have a wide choice of foods but at the same time, due to their increased environmental awareness, they want these products to be environmentally friendly and to respect good farming practices, as well as the welfare of the animals involved. Finally they wish to be informed, and want guarantees of the composition, the nutritional value, the shelf life, the origin and the production methods used. This can be done directly, by means of an efficient labelling system, or indirectly, by checks by public authorities.

Delivering balanced and reliable information to consumers is not a simple matter. Three main complications exist. The first is the difficulty of distinguishing information from advertising. The second related factor is the division of responsibility for informing the consumers between public authorities, private consumer organisations and those attempting, at different levels, to sell to the consumer. Finally there is the usually responsible, but often sensational, influence of the media.

Consumer Expectations

France represents the largest national agricultural and livestock economy in Western Europe. It is also a country with very strong and distinct traditions in food production and consumption. French consumers are highly discriminating and sensitive to issues concerning food. For these reasons, and because the evolution of consumer attitudes in that country have been intensively studied, the French experience post BSE is of particular interest.

As elsewhere, the 1996 announcement on the link between BSE and the vCJD caused a large and sustained reduction in beef purchases from about 180 g per person per week to around 130 g. The development of public attitudes has been debated and examined intensely (Flamant 2001, MAA 2001), as well as stimulating studies in human sciences (sociology, anthropology). A great diversity of behaviour emerged.

Two categories of consumers did not change their habits: those with the highest level of consumption of beef, and those with the lowest level. The former are interpreted as being culturally attached to beef, and prepared to discount perceived risks. The latter, because of low consumption and diversified diet may similarly discount risk. Most of the reduction in individual consumption was due to the behaviour of medium level consumers.

Combris (1997) observed higher reactions in younger people, and concluded that this is evidence of a probable general trend for low consumption of beef in future. Adda (2001) noted that the percent of households making a short term choice to cease beef purchases in France doubled as a result of the crisis. It was also noted that aversive reactions were strongest in Paris and other urban areas least connected to agriculture.

The rolling debate on these issues, and on food in general, "Les Etats Généraux de l'Alimentation", has documented this variety of public attitudes, and concludes that

- official surveillance and guarantees of safety need to be strengthened;
- that these are insufficient in themselves, and that consumers in future will require greater transparency and more information on food sources;
- that local, short chain, supply systems best serve these needs; and
- that these also preserve and promote variety and authenticity in food choice.

Standards

General (general characteristics of a product, with reference to norms such as those of the Codex Alimentarius, the ISO or other internationally accepted norms) and Defined (rules for product processing described in the product specification) Standards can be used efficiently only if they are clearly and simply formulated. The elements therefore that define the standards must be: precisely defined, verifiable by a repeatable procedure, easy to use, and, if possible, cheap. These conditions allow the verification to be reliable and avoid the confusion and arguments, which may arise due to the inclusion of superfluous or misleading elements.

The most frequently used General Standards are those established by the Codex Alimentarius, which are designed to assure the highest levels of consumer health protection and to establish benchmarks for international trade. Nonetheless some aspects, previously overlooked, must be modified to assure consumer safety and quality in every phase of the production cycle. More attention must be paid in the General Standards to the raw materials and the system of production used. The production process must therefore be clearly defined and the products used in farms (animal feed, integrators etc.) must meet defined standards.

Qualitative and quantitative parameters for products must be precisely defined rather than generic descriptions of goals, as is the situation at present. Thus the defined standards must be described in detail, should provide clear information to permit correct and safe use, and, in addition, should include precise guidelines on inspection, sampling and analysis.

Quality assurance

Quality assurance (QA) includes co-ordinated activities including checks on the product and the phases of production to assure that pre-established standards and/or conditions are observed. Respecting these standards and/or conditions guarantees the quality.

Consumer needs can only be guaranteed by adopting quality assurance programs (programs which establish the method, times, figures and costs involved in guaranteeing the application of the activities involved in QA) for farm products (Nardone & Valfrè 1999).

However the needs of the consumer (both the final user and the companies which process farm products) are not limited to food safety. Safety against chemical, physical and microbiological contamination must also be assured as well as the following characteristics:

- sensorial;
- chemical-physical;
- microbiological; and
- technological.

There are many general or sector norms concerning health and hygiene checks and inspections which must be respected for animal food products when raising the animals or processing the product. In addition to these norms greater attention should be paid to the feed of the animals as this is a critical point in assuring the quality of the product and it has not been adequately considered until now.

Today the production of animal feed is regulated to facilitate the free circulation of feedstuff by means of a list of forbidden products or permitted additives. A positive list of feed materials would be the clearest answer to the current lack of definition of feed materials. In the short term, the current negative list needs to be integrated with the positive list of permitted products.

The principles of food safety must be applicable to the feed sector, in particular to clarify the responsibilities of feed producers. With regard to the above, particular situations must be examined and generalisations should be avoided. Here we refer to the proposed regulations on food (Amended Proposal for a Regulation of the European Parliament and of the Council laying down the general principles and requirements of food law, establishing the European Food Authority, and laying down procedures in matters of food safety, COM – 2001- 475 final) which also tend to consider "feed business" *any producer producing, processing or storing feed for feeding to animals on his own holding.*

The effects on quality that the introduction of innovative technology in the production phase has on farms producing typical products must be evaluated when new technology occurs. Action must also be taken with regard to those agricultural practices which may entail risks of contamination (by heavy metals, chemical compounds, mycotoxins, etc.) in growing feed designed for animal consumption. This can be done by formal intervention aimed at increasing the awareness and professional training of the producer. The general principles of hygiene and various Codes of Good Practice must be communicated more widely and also applied in livestock farms.

Thus a strong commitment is necessary until Quality Assurance becomes the norm in all animal husbandry processes. Farmers must be convinced of their key role in Quality Assurance and not see themselves as having only a passive role.

The evolution from a policy of quantity to that of quality which has been seen in the processing and marketing food sectors must also involve primary producers. Management of the systems which assure and document quality requires continuing investment in knowledge of the characteristics of the product and the risk factors which may be present in the productive process used on the farm. This requires involving the workers in the sector and improving their professional training.

To achieve these objectives a policy of technical assistance is essential, aimed at improving the knowledge of the special circumstances both of the farms and the production activity. This will also help to put good production techniques into practice. In this way application of the quality assurance system could also help even small farms to grow.

Great attention must be paid to avoiding duplication of roles which could result in differences in interpretation and conflicts over areas of competence. Training and qualifying farm workers and technical assistants may, in part, offer a valid alternative to adopting the HACCP (Hazard Analysis of Critical Control Points) procedure complex, which is difficult to apply widely in small farms for cost reasons. Involving not only farm workers but also all the others involved in the work of the farm (technical assistants, veterinarians, slaughterers, food processors, feed manufacturers) could result in greater respect for the standards.

3.8 The Place for Regional and Special Quality Products

It is believed that there will be an increase in the demand for traditional and regional products because consumers prefer them to generic products and identify them with positive characteristics. Indeed, consumers often do not trust the modern production methods used in agriculture and believe that production methods linked to a particular area and which use traditional technology are more trustworthy. Thus regional products should be encouraged as they increase consumer trust. Such systems (**Box 9**) also respond very well to other requirements of society, such as sustainability and respect for the environment.

These advantages are recognised in important initiatives of the EU. Regulation (EEC) No 2081/92 lays down common rules which guarantee to producers who respect those rules an exclusive right to use designations of origin or geographical indications entered in the Community register. This avoids unfair competition from "imitation" products while at the same time facilitating the free movement of products which are entitled to the protected designations and indications. It is worth noting that about 550 products have already been registered, of which about 150 are milk products (notably cheeses).

Box 9. Iberian Pig, an Example of Sustainable Animal Production

The production of the Iberian pig and its crosses, particularly with the Duroc-Jersey breed, is a good example of sustainable animal production and an important alternative to conventional systems.

One of the most outstanding breed characteristics is its rusticity that permits good production results. The production is linked to a particular ecosystem called *dehesa*, the result of the traditional interaction among human, animal and Mediterranean forest. The main kinds of trees of this forest are holm oaks and cork trees. The *dehesa* area is distributed mainly in the south-west of Spain and covers about 3 million hectares.

The system is based on the exploitation of natural resources and combines traditional habits and cultural values with specialized modern production systems. The pigs graze freely and eat the acorns produced by the trees. The density of animals is adapted to the available area and no additives are used. The system is therefore considered highly environmental and welfare compatible.

The pigs are slaughtered at 165 kg live weight between 14-15 months old. The meat is mostly used to produce ham and different kinds of sausages, but more and more it is being consumed as fresh pork in restaurants. The meat has a high fat content with high levels of unsaturated fatty acids (55% of oleic acid). Because of this characteristic is considered as a healthy product.

An important and technologically advanced pork industry has developed in the local areas of Iberian pig production and has contributed to strong economic and social development of those regions. In fact, the production of Iberian products represents 10-15% of total pork production in Spain. Iberian ham, the most important, well-known and appreciated Iberian product, because of its special flavour, is sold under a special label and achieves a market price of 30- 40 €/Kg, two to three times more than conventional ham.

Regulation (EEC) No 2082/92 is intended to protect the special features of agricultural or food products which have, independently of their origin, certain characteristics setting them apart from other similar products.

There are, however, two types of problem involved in this:

1) The EC norms only allow the "territorial origin" to be used for the PDO (Protected Designation of Origin) and PGI (Protected Geographical Indication) products. In other cases the EU maintains that citing the production zone of the raw materials used is a barrier to free trade. Meat production has demonstrated the limits of this approach, highlighting the need to trace and describe all phases of production precisely, including the production zone.

2) Until relatively recently, local production systems did not import raw materials from outside, and the whole productive cycle took place in the local area and used only local raw materials. By contrast today the market for raw materials is globalised, and is accessible to small farms which sell only in the local market. Thus regional production *per se* does not meet the demands of the consumer.

PDO and PGI production, governed by EEC regulation 2081/92, are a good example of how these problems can be approached. The geographical origin of these products is recognised and supervised. At the same time product specifications which establish defined standards are designed to protect the consumer and ensure fair competition.

These product specifications define the physical aspect and marketing composition of the final product and define the production methods to be used. For food products of animal origin (meat, processed meat, dairy products) the feeding system for the animals is also normally defined as this is considered a fundamental aspect of the final quality of the product.

Finally the EC regulations which govern PDO and PGI establish that the costs of inspections are paid by the producer as it is considered that the protection given to the product is to their advantage. This is unbalanced in as much as the previous points show that a system of this type is above all of advantage to the consumer. Thus it would be right if not all the costs for inspections to ensure quality fell on the producer.

For typical products the ability to trace their origins and respect for health and hygiene norms is indispensable, as it is for all food products. Thus defined standards must be established for all typical products. This includes defining the elements which make it a typical product, including the territory, as well as the other composition, sensorial, and size parameters, and the principal production phases involved. The raw material used must meet precise standards related to their chemical and microbiological characteristics and the production process involved.

In small farms a distinction must be made between those where the whole production process is carried out with products produced on the farm and those which use raw materials bought elsewhere. In the latter case there must be stringent checks on the composite parameters and the production methods of the raw materials brought in from outside.

These programmes have an importance beyond their economic value: the protection of these designations also raises a question of culture. The defence of these designations is also the defence of the cultural identity of Europe's regions. The system established by Regulations 2081/92 and 2082/92 is undoubtedly one that protects "labels" but behind these "labels" lie products which constitute real "cultural units", each with its own identity and bearing its own history.

Finally, the Commission and the Member States must work within bilateral and multilateral agreements to ensure that PDOs and PGIs are recognised outside the Community. Article 12 of Regulation (EEC) No 2081/92 and Article 22 of the TRIPS Agreement provide a useful starting point for a multilateral registration system for protected designations.

3.9 Organic Production

Organic food production is often proposed as the logical alternative to modern high input farming. Its development depends to a large degree on the increasing consumer demand for safe and healthy food. Although organic foods now account for just 1-2% of retail sales in both the EU and US, expected annual growth in sales is about 20% in both markets (ITC 2002, Lohr 2001). In Europe, some 2% (>144 000) of farms are now certified organic, with an average annual growth in numbers of 25% (Foster & Lampkin 2000).

Land area devoted to organic production in the EU is steadily increasing. Between 1993 and 1998 organic land area went up four fold, from 0.7 million hectares on 29,000 holdings to 2.7 million hectares on 104,000 holdings. This represented 2.1% of the total agricultural area in the EU. Though land in organic systems was below 1% in most countries, it exceeded 5% in Finland and Italy, and reached almost 10% in Switzerland and Austria.

Although organic products are gradually increasing in volume, their overall share of production in the EU remains low, ranging from 0.2% for organic pork to 2.3% for organic fruit. Since EU regulation on organic livestock was introduced only in 2000 data are limited. Available statistics show that the proportion of certified organic livestock in total livestock production is very low (**Table 3.4**). Austria has the highest share of certified organic dairy and other cattle with

Table 3.4. Certified organic livestock and cereals as percent of total production for some European countries (1998) (Source: Foster & Lampkin 2000)

	Cows	Other cattle	Pigs	Sheep	Cereals
Austria	14.7	10.9	1.1	30.4	3.2
Belgium	0.5	0.2	-	1.3	0.2
Germany	1.2	0.9	0.2	4.2	1.4
Denmark	7.0	2.6	0.8	15.7	2.3
Finland	0.7	0.7	0.8	7.3	3.2
France	0.4	0.1	0.1	0.4	0.3
UK	0.2	0.2	0.1	0.1	0.2
Netherlands	0.5	0.2	0.04	0.5	1.5
Sweden	4.3	0.9	0.9	10.4	2.8

10%, whereas in most other countries such production is below 1%. Similarly Austria has the highest proportion of organic pig production (1%) compared to most other EU countries (0.5%), and the highest organic sheep production (30% in Austria, <16% in other EU countries) (Foster & Lampkin 2000).

Organic production has higher costs than conventional production, and therefore requires a price premium. In 2000, the EU average consumer price premiums varied from 31% for organic red wine to 113% for organic chicken. The premium tends to be smaller in countries with well-developed organic production. In Denmark, Austria and Switzerland, consumer price premiums for many organic products were 20% less than the weighted EU average (Hamm *et al.* 2002). This is mainly a consequence of the greater market and the cost-effectiveness of bulk transport and distribution to major retailers in these countries (Michelsen *et al.* 1999). Price premiums for meat and dairy products appeared to be less than for plant products and were in the region of 20-30% for milk and 20-50% for beef and sheepmeat (Kristensen and Thamsborg, 2002). In total, in 2000, organic produce was valued at US$ 7-7.5bn in retail sales in the EU, similar to the US$7.5-8bn sales of organic produce in the US (ITC 2002).

The guidelines for organic agriculture, developed by the International Federation of the Organic Agriculture Movement (IFOAM 1996) have been used to develop the EU regulations on organic agriculture. Following the 1992 CAP reform, most EU member states implemented Council Regulation (EEC) No. 2092/91 defining organic crop production in statutory terms. EU regulation 1804/99, introducing policy on organic animal husbandry and supplementing the existing regulation, was implemented in August 2000, providing and regulating a standard to label food as organic (Rahmann, 2002). Strict requirements are set out in these regulations which must be met before products, whether produced in the EU or imported goods, may be labelled as organic. In particular, compliance must be met in the restriction of the use of synthetic fertilisers, plant pesticides, livestock feed additives and prophylactic antibiotics.

The conversion to an organic production system can take up to three years during which time the principles of organic farming must be followed before products can be considered organic. Losses are often sustained by in-conversion farms. Council Regulation 2078/92 provides financial compensation for losses incurred during this period (Hau & Joaris 2002).

Organic farming aims to provide the consumer with safe food. However, the impact on human health is not known – a Danish investigation found no scientific reliable evidence that organic food ensures better human health (Kristensen and Thamsborg, 2002). Organic farming does provide suitable tools to minimise environmental pollution and nutrient losses at the farm level. By contrast, animal health does not appear to differ significantly between organic and conventional production systems. With regard to animal welfare the higher level of management standards applied in organic based systems provides several requirements for better living conditions of animals. However, there is little evidence for a system-related effect on product quality, which is primarily a function of farm management and is highly variable in both organic and conventional production systems (Sundrum 2001).

3.10 The Place for Science

Much of the development in the livestock sector in the last five decades has been driven by, and indeed made possible by, scientific advances. These have led to great increases in the efficiency of production. This in turn has been essential for the economic and physical sustainability of many different farming systems, as well as being the key to long term reduction in the real cost of food. The ultimate beneficiary of all of these scientific developments is the consuming public.

Science continues to contribute across the full spectrum of the livestock production chain. The result is improved technologies for breeding, feeding, management and health care of animals. In addition, scientific developments are required for improved protection of animal welfare, conservation of genetic resources, management of livestock-environment interaction, efficiency of processing and marketing of livestock products, and to enhance the nutritional and consumer safety aspects of livestock-derived foods.

In the past, most scientific developments were introduced without controversy. If they conferred a benefit, and were economically feasible, they went ahead. Today, these criteria are not enough. New developments must also satisfy increasingly demanding expectations on ethical, safety, welfare and environmental grounds.

Reproductive technologies such as artificial insemination (AI) and embryo transfer (ET) are now mature and accepted parts of the production structure. Practical methods of sex determination by sperm separation are now beginning to be used in commercial practice in cattle breeding. *In vitro* fertilisation (IVF) embryo production is routine. Cloning, including cloning from adult cells, has been achieved experimentally in most species of farm animals. Within the next decade, improved efficiency in these techniques is likely to make them economically feasible, at least in dairy and beef production. These techniques could add considerably to the efficiency of both breeding and production (Cunningham 1999). In addition, freezing of embryos may contribute to the preservation of genetic variability in some species and breeds.

Genetic technology holds the prospect of even greater potential benefits, but could be considerably more controversial. The technical benefit of genetic modification (GM) in plants is now firmly established in such crops as maize, soya bean and cotton. The use of such GM crops has been accepted in the USA and elsewhere, and in 2002 GM varieties accounted for 34%, 75% and 70% of US acreage for these three crops.

Much of the soya bean and corn used in livestock feeding now comes from GM strains. To the extent that these reduce grain production costs, these benefits eventually flow through into reduced feed costs in the livestock chain. More specialised possibilities also exist. Rice has been produced which incorporates a transgene coding for antibacterial proteins. Such grains, when fed to poultry, lead to improved feed conversion ratio without the use of antibiotics.

In the EU, the attitude to GM crops has been cautious. There is widespread public opposition to products from GM plants entering the food chain. In the most recent large scale survey (Eurobarometer 58.0, March 2003) 56% of respondents considered GM food to be dangerous, 71% "do not want this type of food" and 95% want the right to choose. On the basis that the consumer has the right to make an informed choice, this has led to the introduction of labelling regulations. Since 1997 (Regulation no. 258/99) labelling of GM is mandatory.

More recently, opposition has focused on potential environmental effects. The Deliberate Release Directive (2001/18/EC) was implemented in October 2002, bringing improvements to environmental safety assessments and limiting consents to 10 years. However, the European Commission has ruled out a decision on new authorisations for GMOs until Autumn, 2003 at the earliest, following concerns by some member states that the marketing or importation of GMOs might be approved before final EU regulations have been put in place. Most member states consider it would be unsatisfactory to allow commercialisation of GM crops before each individual country has finalised regulations, and some, such as the UK, have yet to enshrine in national laws the EU regulations on GM food, feed, and on the traceability and labelling of GM products. So, at present, the de facto moratorium on marketing consents remains in place.

In the EU, with a much different agro geography to North America, the European Commission (2003) has recognised that the issue of the coexistence of GM, conventional and organic crops is critical. Possible management measures include: isolation distances, buffer zones, pollen barriers, crop rotation, and monitoring regimes. A review of gene flow studies from GM crops, published by the European Environment Agency (2002) concluded that the frequency of gene flow was high from oilseed rape to other oilseed rape and wild relatives; medium to high for sugar beet and low for potatoes, wheat and barley. Maize demonstrates a high frequency of flow to non GM maize, but it has no wild relatives in Europe.

Although a European Directive on liability has been proposed to determine responsibility for damage caused by growing GM crops, it is restricted in scope and currently at an early stage of negotiation. There is currently no EU legislation on economic liability, to protect non GM farmers whose markets might be lost by GM contamination (e.g. licensed organic farmers, whose products are certified GM free by law).

In animals, most of the advances in GM technology have been in mice. In the twenty years since the production of the first genetically altered mouse, more than 1,000 lines of GM mice have been produced for research purposes. In recent years, transgenic pigs, sheep, goats and cattle have been produced. Most of the incentive has been from pharmaceutical interests, seeking to use the animals as bioreactors. Clinical trials using human anti-trypsin and anti-thrombin-3 derived from transgenic sheep are now in progress. Because of high cost, low success rates, and long generation intervals, the development of pharmaceutically useful transgenic lines of livestock is an expensive business. Nevertheless it is likely to be a part of the pharmaceutical industry in the decades to come.

The opportunities for using transgenic livestock in conventional food production are considerably less, again partly because of the high costs involved. In addition, the technology is so far insufficiently addressed. Furthermore, the acceptability of such animals will also be a major issue. Nonetheless, where the objective is improved animal welfare, such objections might be overcome. A good example is the search for transgenic dairy cows with an in-built resistance to mastitis. This is the most expensive disease in the industry, costing US$2 billion per annum in the US. Considerable progress has been made on enhancing mastitis resistance by incorporating into the cow's genome the ability to produce antibacterial enzymes in the udder (Kerr *et al.* 2002). Success in this research would also have the advantage of greatly reducing routine antibiotic use in milk production, a goal already being pursued through conventional methods (**Box 5**).

Apart from directly transforming the genomes of production animals, GM technology can be used in a number of other ways to enhance the efficiency of livestock production and processing. For more than 20 years, most cheese in Europe has been produced using chymosin produced by genetically engineered bacteria. Bovine somatotropin (BST), produced in bacterial culture, is now routinely used to boost milk production in dairy cows in the US. The product is delivered by periodic injection, and results in increased output of the order of 10 - 15%, and increased feed conversion efficiency of 5 - 10%. However, following the recommendations of two expert groups, on the animal welfare (European Commission, 1999a) and public health (European Commission, 1999b) implications of BST use, the EU has banned the commercial use of BST. Even in the USA there are serious concerns over whether this is an economically viable technology. For example, the economic analyses of Tauer (2001) at Cornell University show that at least half the farmers using BST are doing so at a loss, but the complexity of farm systems and inter-year variations in many cases precludes identification of 'winners and losers'. An analysis of BST use, identifying the ethical rationales of its use and non-use, is provided by Mepham (2000).

Less controversial uses of genetic technology lie in its adaptation to improve the efficiency of selection practices. With the development of genetic marker maps, and eventually of whole genome sequence information in all the major species, there are great possibilities for pinpointing genes with beneficial effects on a range of production and health traits. In some cases they can be used to test for, and rapidly eliminate genetic defects, while in others, they can be used to identify animals carrying favourable genes for production or health traits.

The same genetic technologies can also be used for a range of other purposes. The task of documenting genetic differences, and planning and executing genetic conservation programmes can be facilitated by analyses at the DNA level. DNA technologies also offer the ultimate solution to secure animal identification for use in traceability and quality assurance schemes

Scientists have a special role in helping the livestock sector, the public authorities, and society as a whole to find safe and acceptable ways to deal with new technologies. The experience of the BSE crisis has sharpened the perception of these responsibilities. In the BSE crisis, scientists represented all sorts of occupations and interests, including industry employees, Government advisors, representatives of consumer organisations and media commentators. They will continue to be used in this way. Few if any scientists will be completely independent of particular interests. But all speak in the name of science.Preserving the integrity and credibility of scientific advice is important not just for scientists, but for society as a whole. Scientists must therefore accept an obligation in putting any recommendation, to clearly separate the factual basis of such advice from the value judgements which they bring to it. The basis of these value judgements may be financial interest, or personal philosophy on vital values.

Scientists must also recognise the complexity of the context in which such advice may be implemented. This reflects not just the many different interest groups with possibly conflicting objectives, but the particular difficulty of arriving at acceptable trade-offs between gain and risk. For instance, as one example, there is no such thing as *the* precautionary principle: choice of the right level of precaution in different circumstances is a complicated matter involving difficult trade-offs (Jensen, 2002). This, and the fact that scientific advice may vary, are recognised (European Commission, 2000). This Communication states: "Even if scientific advice is supported by only a minority fraction of the scientific community, due account should be taken of their views, provided the credibility and reputation of this fraction are recognised" (7.2) and "Examination of pros and cons cannot be reduced to an economic cost benefit analysis. It is wider in scope and includes non economic considerations" (7.3.4).

References

Adda J. (2001). *Behaviour towards health risks : An empirical study using the CJD crisis as an experiment.* (In preparation, University College London).

Agriculture and Environment Biotechnology Commission. (2001). Crops on Trial. www.aebc.gov.uk

Agriculture and Environment Biotechnology Commission. (2002). Animals and Biotechnology. www.aebc.gov.uk.

Beauchamp T.L. & Childress J.F. (1994). *Principles of Biomedical Ethics* (4th Edition) Oxford University Press, Oxford and New York

Combris P. (1997). L'évolution de la consommation de viande de bœuf depuis 1980. In *Encéphalopathies spongiformes subaiguës transmissibles.* Contribution de l'INRA. 34-38. INRA Editions, Versailles

Cunningham E.P (1999). The application of biotechnologies to enhance animal production in different farming systems. *Livestock Production Science* 58: 1-24

Cunningham E.P. & Meghen C.M. (2001). Biological identification systems: genetic markers. *Revue scientifique et technique, Office International des Epizooties.* 20(2), 491-499.

Curry. (2002). *Farming and Food: A Sustainable Future* by the Policy Commission on the Future of Farming and Agriculture, UK, available from the Cabinet Office, Room LG12, Admiralty Arch, The Mall, London SW1A 2WH, UK or *http://www.cabinet-office.gov.uk/farming*

EU Consumer Policy and Health Protection Directorate. (1996a). Report on Animal Welfare Aspects of the Use of Bovine Somatotrophin, 1999a.

EU Consumer Policy and Health Protection Directorate. (1996b). Report on Public Health Aspects of the Use of Bovine Somatotrophin,(1999b).

European Environment Agency. (2002). Genetically modified organisms (GMOs): the significance of gene flow through pollen transfer. EAA: Copenhagen.

European Commission. (2000). Communication COM(2000)1.

European Commission. (2002). EU the Deliberate Release Directive (2001/18/EC).

European Commission. (2003). GMOs: Commission addresses GM crop co existence, Press Release 5.03.03 http://europa.eu.int).

Flamant J.C. (2001). *A national debate on the food challenges: public perception of animal production and animal products before and during the BSE crisis in France.* EAAP Annual Meeting, Budapest, 22 August, 4 pages

Food Ethics Council. (2001a). *Farming animals for food: towards a moral menu.* FEC, Southwell, Notts, UK.

Food Ethics Council. (2001b). *After FMD: aiming for a values-driven agriculture.* FEC, Southwell, Notts, UK.

Foster C. & Lampkin N. (2000). Organic and in-conversion land area, holdings, livestock and crop production in Europe. *Final Report FAIR3-CT96-1794.*

Hau P. & Joaris A. (2002). Organic Farming. European Commission Report. *http://europa.eu.int/comm/agriculture/envir/report/en/organ_en/report_en.htm*

Hamm U., Gronefeld F., & Halpin D. (2002). *Analysis of the European market for organic food.* Organic Marketing Initiatives and Rural Development. Vol. 1., Aberystwyth.

Hodges J. & Han In K. (Eds). (2000). Livestock, Ethics and Quality of Life (2000). CABI Publishing, Wallingford, Oxon. OX10 8DE, UK. ISBN 0-85199-362-1. HB, pp. 269.

IFOAM. (1996). *International Federation of the Organic Agricultural Movement: Basic Standards For Organic Agriculture and Food Processing,* 10th Edition. SÖL, Bad Dürckheim

ITC, International Trade Centre. (2002). *Overview of world markets for organic food & beverages (estimates).* UNCTAD/WTO.

Jensen K.K. (2002). Moral foundation of the precautionary principle, Journal of Agricultural and Environmental Ethics 15, 59-55.

Kerr D.E, Wellnitz O., Mitra A. & Wall R.J. (2002). *Potential of Transgenic Animals for Agriculture.* 53rd Annual Meeting of the European Association of Animal Production, Cairo, Egypt, 1-4 September 2002.

Kristensen E.S & Thamsborg S.M. (2002). Future European market for products from ruminants. *Organic meat and milk from ruminants.* EAAP publication no. 106. Kyriazakis I & Zervas G. (Eds).

Lohr L. (2001). Factors affecting international demand and trade in organic food products. *ERS/USDA Changing structure of Global Food Consumption and Trade*/WRS-01-1: 67.

MAA. (2001). Etats Généraux de l'Alimentation. Que voulons-nous manger? *Publication Mission d'Animation des Agrobiosciences,* pp. 50

Mepham T.B. (2000). The role of food ethics in food policy. *Proceedings of the Nutrition Society.* 59, 609-618

Mepham T.B. & Crilly R.E. (1999). Bioethical issues in the generation and use of transgenic farm animals. Alternatives to Laboratory Animals 27, 847-855.

Michelsen J., Hamm U., Wynen E. & Roth E. (1999). The European Market for Organic Products: Growth and Development. *Organic Farming in Europe: Economics and Policy* Vol. 7. Stuttgart, University of Hohenheim.

Nardone A. & Valfrè F. (1999). Effects of changing production methods on quality of meat, milk and eggs. *Livestock Production Science* 59:165-182

Netherlands Ministry of Agriculture, Nature Management and Fisheries. (2001). The Future of Dutch Livestock Production -Agenda for Restructuring the Sector. Report to the Ministry.

Phillips N. A., Bridgeman, J. & Ferguson-Smith, M. (2000). *The BSE Inquiry: The inquiry into BSE and variant CJD in the United Kingdom,* Stationery Office, London. *http://www.bse.org.uk/*

Rahmann. (2002). The standards, regulations and legislation required for organic ruminant keeping in the European Union. *Organic meat and milk from ruminants.* EAAP publication no. 106. Editors: Kyriazakis I and Zervas G.

Royal Society. (2001). The use of genetically modified animals.www.roysoc.ac.uk

Sancristobal-Gaudy M., Renand G., Amigues Y., Boscher M.-Y., Leveziel H. & Bibe B. (2000). Traçabilité individuelle des viandes bovines à l'aide de marqueurs génétiques. *INRA, Prod. Anim.,* 13, 269-276.

Schlosser E. (2001). Fast Food Nation. 288 pp. Houghton Mifflin.

Sundrum A. (2001). Organic livestock farming: A critical review. *Livestock Production Science* 67: 207-215

Tauer L. (2001). The estimated profit impact of recombinant bovine somatotropin on New York dairy farms for the years 1994 through 1997. AgBioForum 4, 115-123

Conclusions

This report has been prepared, on behalf of EAAP, by a group of 14 persons, most of whom are scientists involved in and concerned for the European livestock production industry.

In assembling, analysing and interpreting the facts there has been general unanimity. Achieving consensus on the conclusions for the future of the livestock sector has been much less easy. This reflects the varying value judgements of the different members about the broad goals of society, of the sector, and therefore of the report. While the group possesses some expertise in presenting the facts, it claims no special moral authority in setting the goals. These are in any case extremely complex, and involve difficult trade offs between conflicting objectives, as well as between different interest groups.

Behind all this complexity is a major philosophical question: to what extent should future agricultural policy in Europe place food production in a free market context? Historical concerns about food security, and about the social and demographic structure of society, have put agriculture at the centre of EU policy. That policy has been protective of producers. It is now facing substantial change, with commitments to eventual global open competition. The expected benefits for society are chiefly lower food prices. The costs are more diverse, and include reduced incomes for European farmers, and longer, and therefore less transparent, food supply chains. The balance sheet of gains and losses, and of who the beneficiaries and losers are, has been insufficiently quantified and debated.

While the balancing of these interests is a matter for deliberation in the whole of society, policy is eventually crystallised into regulation through the political process. Given, and accepted, that progressively more unrestricted competition is the future, how can valued objectives such as ethical standards in production, authenticity or quality of product, or fair terms of trade be achieved? Since, under the free market, profit maximisation drives all decisions, it seems that these other objectives are unlikely to be served unless the regulatory framework makes them a requirement. Already, substantial change in this direction has taken place to guarantee food safety. A major task for the future is to debate and refine the regulatory context under which the European livestock sector can serve the broad goals of society. A particular challenge for those involved in the sector is to persuade society that food, and the rural environment in which it is produced, have values to the community beyond those of the cash register.

The BSE epidemic, which began in 1986, is now, with high probability, drawing to a close. Though 95% of cases occurred in one country, the economic impact has been felt equally by all beef producers in Europe. Up to 10% of the annual value of beef output has been lost (half through reduced animal value, half in additional costs for control measures). Though the epidemic will, in all probability end, much of the cost and loss will continue indefinitely. In present value terms, it is estimated at €92 billion for the 15 countries of the EU.

The experience of the epidemic has highlighted deficiencies in the production and processing industries, and in the public food safety structures. The dangers in recycling industry waste as feed materials were not appreciated; excessive and opportunistic trading and movement of materials, animals and products was part of the system; identification and traceability were deficient. The response of the public authorities suffered from divided responsibilities, untransparent procedures, insufficient knowledge, and a culture of caution.

Several negative consequences have arisen from these deficiencies. Of prime import has been permanent damage to consumer confidence not just in beef, but in all foods. The reputation of the scientific establishment for providing objective and independent information has been severely downgraded in the public mind. Government authorities have been perceived as protecting sectoral interests rather than the public in general.

Positive outcomes include the wave of corrective measures at national and EU levels, and the establishment of new structures and authorities to bring greater supervision, accountability and integrity to the food chain. These positive developments, while they impose extra costs in the system, costs which will largely fall on primary producers, should be welcomed as necessary and overdue.

Three major unresolved questions remain. The first two concern BSE itself, the origin of which is still not known with certainty, and vCJD in humans, the future of which is also uncertain. The third unresolved issue is the future of MBM. At present all of the 16 million tons of raw material produced each year by the slaughter industry in the EU is rendered and destroyed at a cost exceeding €1 billion. Before BSE it had a protein feed value of more than €0.5 billion. New EU legislation would permit most of this to re-enter the feed industry.

However, despite the strongest of controls and guarantees regarding safety, there is great resistance to such a move. While the origin, presence and transmission of BSE and associated TSEs in animal tissues, food and human bodies remain unknown, no absolute guarantees are possible. A greater influence against implementing such a re-introduction of MBM to the animal feed chain is the resistance of livestock producers rightly fearful of consumer reaction. The only realistic option for the immediate future of this issue is a continuation of the ban on MBM.

The BSE crisis was an unwelcome addition to a list of interrelated challenges already facing the European livestock production sector.

These include:

- Long term decline in real producer prices of about 3% per year.
- Changes in EU policy which will expose producers to increased competition from other areas of the world.
- A growing dependence for economic survival on politically sensitive subsidy programmes, paralleled by a declining influence of producers on policy formation.
- A major power shift in the food chain to dominant retailing and processing firms, further accentuating price pressure on producers.
- Increased costs for enhanced controls and compliance.
- Rapid changes in the pattern of consumer demand.
- Consumer distrust, fed by recurrent food scares, and amplified by a sensitised media.
- As the numbers of producers decline, and as the food chain lengthens and becomes more anonymous, the mutual knowledge and understanding between primary producers and ultimate consumers is reduced.
- A historical structure where three quarters of the 7 million farms in the EU do not have sufficient scale to provide one full-time work and income opportunity.

- The prospect of integrating the 10 million additional farmers in the 10 countries acceding to the EU.
- An intensity of land use in some areas that causes progressive nutrient overloading of the environment.

In the face of these formidable challenges, and energised by the BSE epidemic, European livestock producers, processors and the relevant public authorities have made substantial changes. New food safety agencies have been set up. All cattle and most sheep are identified. Traceability rules are being implemented. New controls on the feed industry have been introduced. Policy at national and EU levels has been adapted.

Many commentators, representing views among producers as well as consumers, feel that these adjustments are not enough. This view, articulated for example in the Curry Report in the UK, The Netherlands' Ministry Report, and in Hodges & Han, 2000, calls for more radical restructuring.

Many of their recommendations are aimed at returning to shorter, more local food chains, rewarding good practice and product quality, and responding to consumer expectations, particularly on safety. The dilemma for producers, policy makers and society is that market forces alone will not deliver these objectives. In particular, it serves the economic purposes of large processing and retailing firms to focus consumer trust on company brands rather than on products identified by region or production system. Companies also need to minimise the costs of these supplies, a goal often best served if their suppliers are producing an undifferentiated product.

The non-monetary values involved in livestock production (safety, ethical production, environmental protection, fair trade, conservation of rural society, respect for tradition, and others) are important. However, it is quite ineffective to simply advocate respect for these values. They will be respected only if it is profitable to do so, or there are penalties involved in not doing so. In the context of this report it is not possible to describe or invent all the mechanisms required, but the general point is that it requires either profit or regulation. As the market is now evolving, profit is king. If the non-monetary values are to be respected, the free market needs to be circumscribed by formal requirements. The task for the future is to develop these so that they achieve their objective, without simply serving the interests of particular groups or increasing the burden of regulation to unreasonable levels.

Producers, processors or retailers are all most responsive if desirable practice is profitable and undesirable practice carries penalties. It is therefore important to emphasise the necessity of ensuring that public policy, through its standards and regulations, acknowledges and protects the non-monetary values which are part of the food production system. As a result of BSE, this is now well recognised for food safety. Similar initiatives are needed to define the standards of ethical production, environmental protection, and fair trade within which the market must operate.

While the broad evolution of the marketing structure is not favourable to these goals, there are many examples of how producer groups are working together with retailers to provide, and be rewarded for, quality products. This provides one model for recognising and supporting genuine differentiation in production. Already, the PDO and PGI systems, and certification for organic producers, are in place.

Another model is where the producers invest collectively in processing and distribution. This also already exists and is very effective in much of the EU dairy industry and in the pigmeat sector in Denmark. Such large co-op structures can strike a fair balance between the interests of the producers and other actors in the food chain, and are perhaps the best way of re-establishing the connections that have been weakened. The livestock sector should value and continue to invest in the co-operative structures that have served European society well for over a century.

In all countries and at the EU level, legal constraints can be invoked where a dominant market position could lead to unfair trading practices or reduced competition. There is evidence (e.g. in UK) that dominant retail groupings exploit their strength to impose unreasonable terms on their suppliers. Given the pace of which food retailing (and processing) power is being concentrated, there is a strong case for closer monitoring and control of such abuse of economic power.

The question of food safety should not be an issue in the competitive market: all food should be safe. Some companies may wish to add to their customers' sense of security by adding guarantees, testing regimes and traceability above what is required by law. However, the basic safety certification of food and its production systems should be the responsibility of public agencies.

The failures which led to the BSE crisis have provided a hard lesson for all involved in the European livestock sector. A technical innovation (use of MBM), which had been judged safe, and had been widely used for more than 40 years, proved to be the instrument which spread a new and frightening disease in animals and humans. All scientific innovation is now suspect. This has strengthened public opposition to developments such as GM crops, use of BST in milk production, or growth promoters in meat production. Producers are often ambivalent – appreciating the technical advantages, but unsure on long term safety and public reaction. Policy is driven mainly by these wider public attitudes. Present EU policies do not allow these technologies to be used. As evidence on food safety and other concerns accumulates, and as public attitudes change, these policies may also evolve. Livestock producers must work within these regulations. They must also recognise that Europe has chosen a deliberately cautious path, and that though they are precluded from taking advantage of some technical developments, this can be offset by increased consumer appreciation of and loyalty to local products.

Beyond the many difficulties which have followed from or been exacerbated by the BSE crisis, the European livestock sector has a fundamental problem of the scale of individual enterprises. Too many farms are too small to provide an income for one person. This structural problem will be made more acute by the continuous price reductions which will flow from the progressive globalisation of trade in agriculture. This is a problem for which there is no direct solution. Unit scale is increasing, but, as can be seen in USA, scale alone does not assure economic survival.

The inevitable further decline in numbers engaged in livestock production, and the parallel increase in scale of remaining production units, has no particular end point. It is a continuing process, shared by other sectors in an evolving world economy. For Europe, it leads to a spectrum of structures, varying greatly across the continent, but increasingly classifiable into two groups:

- efficient, full time, larger units, responsible for most of production, but representing a small fraction (at present one quarter) of producers
- smaller, part time, units, managing a high proportion of land, but only partially reliant on agricultural production for income.

EU policy is being adapted rapidly to meet the needs of society, and of these different sectors of production. The challenge is to manage change in a fair and balanced way, driven primarily by Europe's own requirements, and recognising that measured change, rather than stasis or abrupt adaptation can bring greatest benefits at least cost.

Despite the problems created by continuous adaptation, and by occasional crises such as BSE, the European livestock sector has a very positive future for many of its actors. Its strengths include:

- A well endowed resource base, with good climates and soils, well capitalised farms, and well developed services.
- A highly skilled workforce, mainly independent owners, with deep traditions of good husbandry, and with well developed organisational structures.
- A large internal market of 478 million, which takes 95% of its production, and appreciates its products.
- A common agricultural policy, through which measured change and progress can be made.

Acronyms

ACP: African, Caribbean and Pacific Countries

AGP: Antimicrobial Growth Promoters

AI: Artificial Insemination

BSE: Bovine Spongiform Encephalopathy

BVD: Bovine Virus Diarrhoea

CAP: Common Agricultural Policy of the EU

CEEC: Central and Eastern European Countries

CJD: Creutzfeldt-Jakob Disease

CSF: Classical Swine Fever

DEFRA: Department for the Environment, Food and Rural Affairs, (UK)

DSSP: Degree of Soil Saturation with Phosphorous

EAGGF: European Agricultural Guidance and Guarantee Fund

EFPRA: European Fat Processors and Renderers Association

EFSA: European Food Safety Authority

ERS: Economic Resource Service, (USA)

ET: Embryo Transfer

EU: European Union

FAO: Food and Agriculture Organization of the United Nations

FDA: Food and Drug Administration, (USA)

FEC: Food Ethics Council, (UK)

FMD: Foot and Mouth Disease

FSIS: Food Service Inspection Service, (USA)

GATT: General Agreement on Tariffs and Trade

GDP: Gross Domestic Product

GM: Genetically Modified

GMO: Genetically Modified Organism

HACCP: Hazard Analysis of Critical Control Points

IBR: Infectious Bovine Rhinotracheitis

IFIA: International Fertiliser Industry Association

ISO: International Standard Organization

IVF: *In Vitro* Fertilization

LDC: Less Developed Countries

MBM: Meat and Bone Meal

MRM: Mechanically recovered meat

NPV: Net Present Value

OECD: Organisation for Economic Co-operation and Development

OFT: Office of Fair Trading, (UK)

OIE: Office International des Epizooties

PDO: Protected Designation of Origin

PGI: Protected Geographical Indication

PMWS: Postweaning Multisystemic Wasting Syndrome

PSE: Producer Support Estimate

QA: Quality Assurance

SEAC: Spongiform Encephalopathy Advisory Committee, (UK)

SRM: Specified Risk Material

TGE: Transmissible Gastro-Enteritis

TSE: Transmissible Spongiform Encephalopathies

USDA: United States Department of Agriculture

vCJD: variant Creutzfeldt-Jakob Disease

WTO: World Trade Organisation

Printed in the United States
by Baker & Taylor Publisher Services